Allison's story is a real insight into her search for a way to help the body heal itself from the very rare cancer she battled, while still being a wife and a mother and going through life's challenges.

Medical cannabis was a very taboo subject when Allison and I first met. She was cautious to open up to me about it but I'm glad she did. Her knowledge through experience is now my knowledge to pass onto my clients who may go through something similar. Allison's book will make you a little teary and also give you a chuckle.

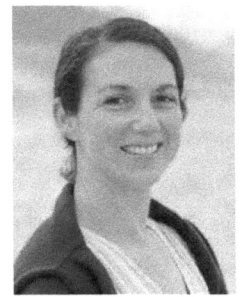

Thank you, Allison, for sharing this with us. This in itself shows what a caring person you are.

Naomi San Jose
Aust. Reg. Remedial Massage Therapist

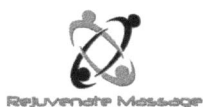

Terminal to Remission with Cannabis Oil draws you in from the beginning and keeps you hooked till the end. It makes a heavy subject light and easy to understand, personalising it with little wisps of humour and irony. It's a story that needs to be told.

Gail Hester
Founding member Medical Cannabis Users Association of Australia Inc
Secretary Legalise Cannabis Party NSW
Registered Office Legalise Cannabis Australia Party

I moved into the street where Allison lives as she was in the middle of her cancer journey. I remember the day she told me that she had about two years to live and I was horrified that this wonderful, tough, warm-hearted person whom I had just met was facing such a harsh, brief future, leaving John and Nathan to continue on without her.

In this book, Allison leads us deep into her life, her family, her work and home-making and achieving her personal goals. She then describes the misery of her cancer and standard medical treatment followed by her extraordinary search for a more humanistic form of treatment.

This wonderfully honest book is about determination and courage and will inspire anyone facing an impossible life hurdle.

Jane Shamrock
Retired Occupational Therapist
GDipOT MA PhD (Sunshine Coast)

Thanks for sharing this very personal account. You have been through so much and come out the other side. Well done for having such a strong attitude and sharing your inspirational story.

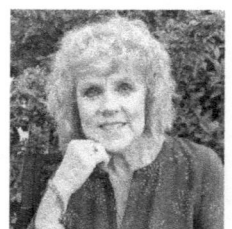

Lucy Haslam
Founder of United in Compassion
(Australia's peak medical cannabis advocacy body)
Retired Registered Nurse

Allison has coherently and affectionately documented those difficult years living with her cancer. Not just once but on three occasions, she has questioned, argued, cried and battled her way to the finish line, always with her family as her priority. Allison was told her life would end, yet she is still living and has bravely shared the horrendous illness she suffered, the many operations, treatment, doubt and lack of support from others, and eventually her final success to remission.

Cannabis was her friend, her saviour and that lifeline for which she searched. I'm so glad she found it and can share her 'no holds barred' book with you all. *Terminal to Remission with Cannabis Oil: An Australian success story* will not fail to inspire and motivate the reader and reinforce that the medical profession, on occasion, does not always have the answers.

I am immensely proud of the woman I met many years ago and even prouder of my friend and author of this amazing, insightful book. Read it, enjoy it, learn from it, and please pass it on to your nearest and dearest, as Allison reminds us that life is precious and to never give up hope.

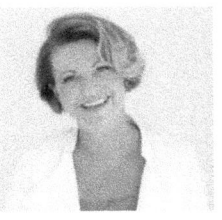

Shelagh Brennand
Retired Police Inspector
Former Stroke Ambassador
Author of A Stroke of Poetry

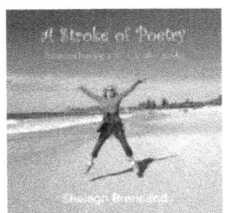

In her book, Allison has presented her life's journey, highlighting all that is good about medical cannabis and all that is wrong with the current system that controls the supply under irrational government regulations.

Cannabis was initially described as a dangerous drug with no medical uses but has now been revealed as the only completely non-toxic medical drug in current use, with a positive impact on an exceptionally broad range of afflictions, acting through the endocannabinoid system.

Allison's perilous cancer journey was made more hazardous by a lack of quality testing of the cannabis products that were helping to extend her life.

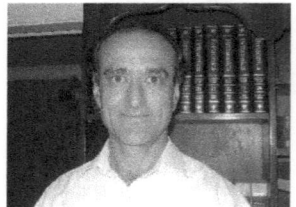

Dr Andrew Katelaris
MB BS (Syd) MD (UNSW)

Terminal to Remission with Cannabis Oil

An Australian success story

Allison McMaster

Dedicated to Mum and Dad, who are in another place, and those who have since passed or are fighting for their lives

Terminal to Remission with Cannabis Oil: An Australian success story
Author – Allison J. McMaster

© Allison J. McMaster, 2023
www.terminaltoremissionwithcannabisoil.com.au
info@terminaltoremissionwithcannabisoil.com.au
PO BOX 6058, Mooloolah Valley QLD 4553

This book details the author's personal experiences with and opinions about collecting duct carcinoma and the use of medicinal cannabis oil. The author is not a healthcare provider. This book is not intended as a substitute for consultation with a licensed healthcare practitioner, such as your physician. Before you begin any healthcare program or change your lifestyle in any way, you should consult your physician or another licensed healthcare practitioner to ensure that you are in good health and that the examples contained in this book will not harm you.

The statements made are not intended to diagnose, treat, cure, or prevent any condition or disease. Please consult with your own physician or healthcare specialist regarding the suggestions and recommendations made in this book.

Except as specifically stated in this book, neither the author nor publisher, nor any authors, contributors or other representatives will be liable for damages arising out of or in connection with the use of this book. This is a comprehensive limitation of liability that applies to all damages of any kind, including (without limitation): compensatory, direct, indirect or consequential damages; loss of data, income or profit; loss of or damage to property and claims of third parties.

This book provides content related to physical and/or mental health issues that have been experienced by the author, and the events and situations depicted within are a true representation of how the author perceived these events. As such, use of this book implies your acceptance of this disclaimer.

All rights reserved. This book may not be reproduced in whole or part, stored, posted on the internet, or transmitted in any form or by any means, electronic, mechanical, photocopying, recording, or other, without permission from the author of this book.

Editing, design and publishing support by www.AuthorSupportServices.com

ISBN: 9781922375230

A catalogue record for this book is available from the National Library of Australia

Foreword

Allison had already been diagnosed with a rare cancer when I met her in 2015. It is said that a terminal diagnosis can have a profound effect on a person, in that they often take extra joy in little things that others may take for granted – a blue sky or a blooming flower – and that they don't sweat the small stuff. In this respect many people fundamentally change. Of course, the fear of death and the unknown adds a heaviness. Death is such a sanitised subject in western countries because of the intangibility of what happens spiritually. Death reprioritises life and Alli had embraced that.

Through the work with my charity My Wedding Wish, where we gift weddings to the terminally ill, I deal with many people who have had a terminal prognosis. I'm always aware of the nuances of each person and am awed by the tenacity and drive to live. When I met Alli, she shone like sunshine. Her laugh and her down to earth personality made her easy to like. Then one day she asked if we could meet for a coffee. "Will you conduct my funeral?" she asked and then explained she wanted to get everything in order so the onus didn't fall on her husband. Alli spoke about her fears for her son and his future – life was heavy for her that day. Yet still we laughed. I said, "Of course I will, but let's talk about it when you're a bit closer." I didn't think planning her funeral would be a productive use of our time at that point. She'd already started taking the cannabis oil and she looked great. The funeral plans could wait.

And now, with Alli in remission, I'm so thrilled that those funeral plans will take a back seat as she takes her life by the horns and enjoys the ebb and flow of her world. Alli's book is her journey to healing, which of course is why she wrote it in the first place – to give hope to those in otherwise hopeless situations.

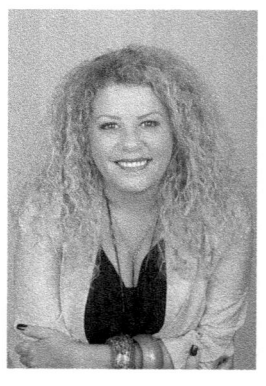

Thank you, Alli, for documenting your journey to health and sharing it with the world. I pray it changes lives and becomes a guide to health for many.

Dr Lynette Maguire
Researcher, Author, Speaker – Now Generation
CEO, Founder – My Wedding Wish Ltd.

Contents

Foreword	v
Prologue – Nimbin	1
"It's a rare cancer"	5
Growing up in the 80s	15
Building a family	19
Becoming a mum	27
Finding fitness	37
The big move	43
The symptoms	57
The treatment	65
Preparing to say goodbye	79
What are the odds?	85
It's the green I need	87
Making memories	107
Pleading with a drug dealer	125
Safety first	131
My Wedding Wish	135
My bestie and unlikely friends	141
Unwelcome returns	147

Mental health roller coaster	161
Smoking the stigma	179
Epilogue – Moving on	199
About the author	205
Acknowledgements	207
Additional resources	209
References	211

Prologue – Nimbin

August 2014

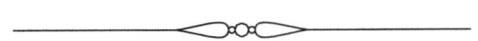

It was a long time ago that I visited this town. I was in my late teens and loved adventure. Although I was more of a drinker than a pot smoker, Nimbin was a place where you could feel free and learn anything to do with growing, eating or smoking cannabis. It had a reputation. And things had not changed in the many years since I had last visited this community of peace-loving, alternative townsfolk – it was a place where you could easily acquire herbs of any description. And the best place to 'score pot'.

I never imagined I would be the one in this position. I needed to score. I never for a moment thought I would think – let alone write – about it and share my story with the world. But as I walked tentatively along the damp, moss-covered back streets of the small community of Nimbin in New South Wales, it was the only thing on my mind.

I was already living on borrowed time. The possibility I could buy more of it through one of the characters who lined the alleyways was the only thing propelling my feet forward, one in front of the other, despite my inner terror of the unknown. Fear of being busted during the transaction by undercover police, fear of being robbed or, worse still, being met with foul play, although highly unlikely, filled my mind. Making a drug deal was not something I would do on a regular basis in my normally very average lifestyle.

> *Making a drug deal was not something I would do on a regular basis.*

I was slightly more confident because my husband John was only a few steps behind me. I knew he would go to the ends of the earth for me if it meant we could stay together for even a month longer. It turned out that we only had to drive three-and-a-half hours from our Sunshine Coast home. However, we decided to trek the back way, which would be less conspicuous. The fear of being pulled over by police was real. Having my son remember me for being a drug-convicted mother was not something I wanted. So, the trip was an hour longer. It was more treacherous in our motorhome on wet, windy roads. It was petrifying. I felt like we were snails lumbering along with our cumbersome shell on our backs.

Just twelve months earlier, I had been told I was going to die before my time. The stony-faced doctor looked me in the eye and told me to spend my last year wisely. "Go on holidays, enjoy life, make memories." It seemed like simple advice, but I wasn't prepared to go without a fight.

My body had been invaded by collecting duct carcinoma, a rare kidney cancer that statistically usually affects the unfit, obese, smoking, alcohol-drinking male over seventy.

Prologue – Nimbin

I was only forty-six. It wasn't fair. I was fit and healthy. I took care of myself. I did everything right. But this was my new unwelcome reality.

Traditional treatments – chemotherapy and radiation – had wreaked havoc on my body, but I never questioned their validity. I wanted to make sure I did everything I could to prevent cancer from coming back. When I first heard about cannabis oil, I laughed, thinking my husband was pulling my leg as he piped up with all of this knowledge. A look at his face quickly told me he was serious.

I had nothing to lose. Literally nothing.

I was knocking on death's door, and if someone told me consuming dog shit would cure me, I would have eaten it. Cannabis oil, although a big unknown for me at the time, seemed like a much more pleasant option.

The only catch was that it was illegal in Australia at the time. I was dicing with my freedom and the possibility I could spend my remaining months in jail if I was caught with the very thing that I hoped would prolong my life.

As a newly enrolled nurse with a strong sense of morals and ethics, this signalled the start of a somewhat dual existence for me. One where I had to rely on underground channels to get access to medicinal cannabis oil to help me manage terminal cancer while remaining the same sensible woman to the outside world.

> *I was dicing with my freedom.*

I'm on a mission to empower cancer victims with knowledge. I was challenged in so many ways throughout my journey, encountering personal obstacles and mental tests. With the help of my support team, I found strength in my relationships. I also found power and confidence within myself, and this has helped me conquer the nightmare I was living through.

I'm on a mission to empower cancer victims with knowledge.

Now I feel the need to share my journey to help empower others who may be going through the same or a similar ordeal. Information leads to knowledge. Knowledge leads to empowerment. With empowerment, decisions that are right for you can be made.

Armed with knowledge, you will be able to make an informed decision about whether medicinal cannabis oil is right for you.

"It's a rare cancer"

4 August 2013

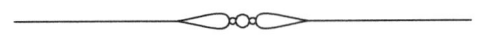

I don't know if I was shivering because the room was so cold or because my nerves were wreaking havoc on my body. It was both. Anyone who has been in the in-between room where they prep you for surgery just before you go into the operating room knows this awful feeling.

This is real. This is a life and death situation. This may be the last time I see my family.

The pill the surgical team gave me slowly started to work its magic and helped me to stop worrying so much. My nerves and my racing mind slowly eased. My mind had been filled with sad thoughts. I told the staff how I was missing my father's funeral because of the operation I was about to

> **This may be the last time I see my family.**

endure. It was all I could think about. I requested the date of the funeral be moved so I could attend, but this was deemed impossible. Changing the operation was not an option either. As anyone who has relied on the public hospital system knows, there was a risk I would be put at the back of the waitlist if I didn't go ahead with my surgery. And here I was, about to be wheeled into the operating theatre while the rest of my family was saying goodbye to Dad. He had lost his battle with both prostate and lung cancer a week earlier.

The staff looked at each other without expression then at me. They wheeled me into an even colder room where I took a deep breath and let out a sigh as I prepared my mind and my body to be hammered by the surgery I was about to undergo.

"You'll doze off very soon," the surgical assistant murmured as he held the anaesthetic mask up to my face. I was instructed to count backwards from ten. *My worries are not their worries*, I reasoned. I have blurred memories of thinking about my dad and not being at his funeral. In my state, I felt that he would understand. I thought about my late mum watching over and protecting me as I drifted off to sleep on the surgeon's table. I hoped my parents did not need me to come to them in the afterlife yet. I hoped they would realise that Nathan, my son, needed me more here on earth, as did John, my husband.

In a matter of seconds, there were no worries at all.

In what seemed like the amount of time it takes for someone to click their fingers, a soft voice said my name. I was so confused. I thought it was Mum repeating my name. But I realised the medication was playing tricks on me as my mum passed away in 1999. When the nurse repeated my name again, I realised where I was.

I slowly opened my eyes, just enough to be blinded by the glaring lights in the clinical setting, with monitors repeatedly beeping and alarms going off. *I don't want to wake up.* The sleep

I was having was the best I'd had in a long time. But the nurse standing next to the bed kept repeating my name. It became very annoying. I tried to turn my back to her, to try to reclaim that peaceful sleep I had been enjoying. Then the pain hit. *I've had surgery.* It took my brain a few seconds to catch up with what my body knew.

I heard soft voices again. Only these were familiar. My husband, John, and thirteen-year-old son, Nathan, were standing at my bedside, talking quietly. I turned my head towards them and managed a small smile. Nathan asked when I was coming home. I was too groggy to reply. John smiled back at me while patting Nathan on the back in a reassuring way. I was so relieved that I had actually woken up. I was back in the real world. *Mum and Dad hadn't needed me yet after all.* The thought made me breathe a sigh of relief. I didn't die. I have more time.

My kidney and the tumour that had seized hold of it were successfully removed, but the first couple of days in the hospital were still very hard. John and Nathan visited me every day, but they could never stay long as Nathan became 'bored' – it was one of his dominant autism traits. John was getting visibly annoyed with Nathan's behaviour as he kept asking about all the machines that were connected to my body. John tried to ask how I was feeling, but Nathan made it hard to have a normal conversation. I tried to move to reposition myself and groaned again. John was able to establish how much pain I was in by my facial expressions. I had forgotten to push the button

> *I didn't die. I have more time.*

beforehand, the one that gave me a hit of morphine to numb the pain.

Nathan kept asking if I was okay. I kept reassuring him. I didn't need to concern him. John knew my pain was present and often unbearable but was relieved when the drugs kicked in and I stopped grimacing. It wasn't long before I was able to mask my true feelings and assume my usual happy self.

John could see I was exhausted and wanted to sleep. I didn't mean to nod off while he was talking to me, but that's what I did. I said my goodbyes as they left. The medications had a hold on me.

The next two nights were horrible. I was put in a ward with five old, snoring men. I couldn't understand why the medical team had done this. I soon realised it was the urinary ward. I couldn't sleep properly unless I drugged myself up. All the men in this ward had urinary issues and here was I, the only female and easily two decades younger than the rest of them. The sound coming from the ward must have sounded like a freight train, times five.

One day after waking up from a light sleep, the group of women who had started off as my fitness clients and quickly become great friends of mine were standing together at the end of my bed. They were talking together when I saw them. They were trying to be quiet. I think I heard one of them say loudly, "Be quiet!!" I smiled broadly. I didn't think it possible for these women not to have something to giggle about. They had taken the time to come and visit me and I perked up a lot as they distracted me with their chatter. I told them that the night before, a nurse kindly came over to my bed and covered my exposed breast with the sheet. I was twisted up in the cotton nightgown and, unknowingly, had not concealed it under the many layers of cotton.

On the third day, John came without Nathan. My son didn't want to come. He had decided hospitals weren't nice places and he didn't like seeing me the way I was. I was okay with that. I understood his reasoning and never doubted his love. At my request, John also brought earplugs for me. Sleep deprivation was being added to the aches and pains associated with my surgery and recovery, and I hated it, so I was beyond relieved when the nurses offered me a bed in the treatment room. This room could hardly fit the single bed. I found it amusing. I was squeezed in among all the medical supplies and observation machines, but at least I could finally get a much better night's sleep.

I rang one of my sisters on her way to work because I felt I needed her emotional support. She came but said she could not stay long as she had many cleaning jobs to complete that day. The three of us were making small talk when five specialists squeezed into the room. The man at the front of the group told me the surgery had been successful and they had removed the entire tumour along with my left kidney.

They were concerned, however, that the tumour was a cancer, but they weren't sure what type it was. I felt a 'told you so' moment when they said this. My sister had reasoned that I was a hypochondriac and had fobbed me off whenever I mentioned my health.

"It isn't something we've seen before," the specialist said matter-of-factly.

"We have taken a sample and will get a biopsy and send it overseas to get the type of cancer confirmed. Then we can look at treatment options," one of them informed me. I felt somewhat disconnected from my body as this news was being delivered. This was all so surreal. *Is this actually happening to me?* But knowing that more and more people survive cancer with modern treatments, I felt confident I would survive too. I also felt a slight relief that my sister was there to hear this news first-hand. She had previously doubted the seriousness of my situation. Now it was laid out by medical professionals in a way she could not fob off.

> *This was all so surreal.*

Each day, I could see an improvement in each of the tasks I managed to accomplish, and the day after the meeting with the specialists, I was allowed to go home. Waiting for the urology specialist's appointment, when I would hear the news of the cancer type, took another two months. I can easily say it was the most unsettling period of my life. I had no control over anything and simply had to wait.

While I was in this torturous limbo of uncertainty for sixty days, I accepted the fact I had cancer and would probably follow the usual pathway to survival: a treatment of chemotherapy or radiation and whatever complementary drugs I needed to take to make sure we annihilated it.

I felt hope that medical advances were happening all the time and survival rates for the cancers I knew – breast, lung, prostate – were all on the rise as research advanced treatment options.

"It's a rare cancer"

The day of the urologist appointment arrived and I was beyond nervous as I waited for the news. I had played out so many scenarios in my head. Everything from, "Oh, we are so sorry! We were wrong, there is no cancer," all the way through to, "We still don't know what type of cancer you have." Thoughts like these can do weird things to the mind.

It turned out they did have a definitive answer, but it was nothing I could have imagined myself.

"Collecting duct carcinoma," the specialist said to me as he looked up from his notes.[1] "But we will have to double-check the results."

He may as well have been talking another language. I had no idea what he had said and asked him to give me a copy of the report and write the name down on it as there was no chance I would walk away from the appointment and remember its name.

"It is a rare and aggressive form of cancer and you are not the typical patient. It usually presents in males. The median age is sixty-three. It's a very nasty type of cancer to have and the prognosis is not great, statistically speaking. Twelve months... two years at best..."

> *It is a rare and aggressive form of cancer.*

He kept talking, but it was all so overwhelming that I felt like it wasn't real. My mind was repeating the words 'rare... aggressive... twelve months'. I was not listening to much else. I felt like I was in a movie of some sort. He wasn't talking to me. *He was mistaken...*

he had to be. The seriousness of what I was up against hit home when he referred me to see an oncologist and I was scheduled to start chemotherapy treatment the following week.

I came home from the hospital and couldn't get out of the car in the driveway. The tears flooded my cheeks as I cried my heart out. *This isn't true! This can't be real. How could this happen to me? I just got my nursing diploma! I'm not ready for this! My family needs me. Nathan needs me.* So many thoughts, feelings, emotions... all colliding in my head. I felt cheated. I'd just got to my prime in life and had never felt better. Now the foundations I had thought were so solid were beginning to crumble. A massive headache came on from the crying, and my eyes were red and puffy. I could hardly see as my eyelids were so inflamed. My sinuses kept flowing and I could hardly breathe.

> *Cancer doesn't happen to people like me. It happens to other people.*

Despite the doctor warning me not to, I searched the internet for information on the cancer I had. In everything I read about patients with my cancer, the outcome was that they died within two years. In research reported by *Cancer Management and Research*, the scientist concluded the overall one-, two- and five-year survival rates were 45.5%, 36.4%, and 8.8% respectively.[2] The median survival time was eleven months. I don't regret doing my own research as I didn't want to be left in the dark about anything.

I didn't want to believe it. *Cancer doesn't happen to people like me. It happens to other people.* People who don't look after *themselves, like my mum and dad, who smoked and drank alcohol on a daily basis. Those years of changing my life around – giving up cigarettes, losing weight, becoming a mentor for others – were all for nothing.*

I learned that stage four is the most serious stage of cancer. In stage four, the cancer is advanced or metastatic, meaning it has spread to other parts of the body.[3] While my tumour was within the kidney, it had also spread to several lymph nodes around the kidney and it was definitely aggressive, meaning it could grow and spread quickly.[4] This worried me no end. It annoyed me when people thought, because I had kidney cancer, it must be like getting a tooth pulled out! It's in the kidney, so if you just remove the kidney, the cancer is all gone, right?

The Cancer Council estimates that more than 4,500 people in Australia were diagnosed with kidney cancer in 2022, and it remains much more common in men.[5] The risk of being diagnosed by age eighty-five is one in sixty-five. The five-year survival rate for kidney cancer is 78.5%.

However, collecting duct carcinoma (CDC) accounts for less than 1% of all renal cancers.[6] And the prognosis was frightening to say the least. This was *not* the way I wanted to be special in life. I looked at the risk factors of kidney cancer and shuddered at the first few: smoking and workplace exposure to asbestos or cadmium.[7] *Maybe working in that factory with asbestos linings in the guards of the machinery was the culprit. It's something I will never know. It wouldn't make any difference.*

> **This was not the way I wanted to be special in life.**

We all signed waivers for the firm's liability if we got cancer or any other disease.

The rest of the factors were not applicable to me: overuse of pain relievers containing phenacetin – non-steroidal anti-inflammatory (NSAIDs) – for example, medications with ibuprofen; a family history of kidney cancer; being overweight or obese; high blood pressure; and being male.

The oncologist explained to me there was no real known way to treat this cancer, but the chemotherapy drugs he was going to give me were the same drugs used for bladder cancer. According to the oncologist, this was best practice. So, I decided to follow what was prescribed by the people who knew what they were doing, because they were the professionals with years of experience. I hoped it would be enough to save me.

Growing up in the 80s

1982

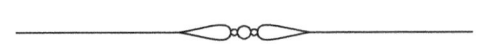

I grew up in Sale, Victoria. In the eighties, everyone smoked cigarettes and the occasional joint or bong and drank alcohol. I thought this was a normal part of being a teen. I partied hard but never really liked smoking pot. I had tried it a few times but felt I didn't have control of my own behaviour. I didn't like the high it gave me and didn't like putting myself in vulnerable situations, being a young teenage girl. My preferred substances of abuse were alcohol and cigarettes... lots of cigarettes... a packet a day. Sometimes two packets if I was clubbing. When I was at school, if I wasn't wagging, I was able to save my school lunch money to buy the packets for the weekend's activities.

I figured cigarettes couldn't be that bad because both of my parents smoked. Mum was a nurse. I thought, *Surely, she wouldn't do things to harm herself.* But the risks weren't known back then. Smoking was promoted as being sexy and an intelligent decision to make. Of course, we all know now that's not the reality.

I had lots of friends to drink with, so when I was sixteen, I would usually be pissed all weekend. In Sale, this was the thing to do. I was no good at sports, although I tried many different types and cost my mother the earth. I felt like there was nothing else to do.

My parents felt I was out of control. I know they had no idea how to 'tame' me. On one occasion, my mum took me down to the police station to get them to talk some sense into me. Some weekends I would sneak out of the house when everyone else was in bed. I was rebellious and not very nice as a teen. I guess we all go through some form of rebellion or another. This was mine.

At the time, I was a little resentful about my parents not supporting me in my choice of career. I wanted to be a DJ. They thought it was a ridiculous idea. Perhaps it was. Female DJs in the 80s were unheard of. I hated the fact that every opportunity for some kind of career meant having to move to the city. Because I was so shy, this did not seem like it was an option at all. A DJ was a perfect job. I loved music and I could hide behind a radio microphone all day. One DJ friend even said I had the perfect face for radio. It went over my head at the time. But I now know he was just trying to be funny.

Casting aside my dream of radio announcing stardom, I worked at a factory in Sale. As I became more mature and confident, I felt the need to cut ties with the country and transferred to a factory in Melbourne in the early nineties. From then, it was factory work, factory work and more factory work.

I always dreamed of making something of myself. I loved Australian comedy and shows like *Fast Forward* and *The*

Comedy Company. I told myself, *One day I am going to write for a show like that.* Political correctness has changed all that now. What used to be hilarious then is not so funny anymore.

While working in the factories on afternoon shift, I studied to be a writer, achieving my Diploma of Professional Writing and Editing. Even though nothing came of it at the time, I believe things happen for a reason. It was many years in the making, but the result of that study is this book.

Thankfully, I settled down a little while living in Melbourne. I still liked a drink or ten. I still liked going to see bands on the weekend and going to Darby's Disco in Caulfield. I used to love partying with my sisters. We had such great times.

I used to love partying with my sisters.

My parents moved to a smaller country town in Victoria for their retirement years. A quiet, simple life. No big bills, which came with the larger country town I grew up in. No worries about neighbours being on the doorstep or giving Dad 'the shits'.

I remember Mum being sick for most of my childhood. She survived bowel cancer. She was diagnosed with it while I was in high school. I am almost ashamed to say it, but at the time I was more concerned about boys and what my weekend plans were. Her surgery was brutal and I didn't realise the colostomy bags that came in a package in the mail were a private thing that Mum was really embarrassed about. I didn't understand the seriousness of my mum's illness. She never told us anything and I didn't ask. But through my nursing studies, I now understand.

When Mum announced that the cancer had come back in 1998, she knew she was not going to be so lucky this time. It had appeared in her pancreas. This was the beginning of the end.

Much later in life, Dad would become a victim of prostate cancer. He was not one to go to the doctors "because they only tell you there is something wrong". He became frail very quickly, but I will always recall him being such a trooper. Before that, he never caught so much as a cold and I believed he would pull through this as well.

Building a family

October 1995

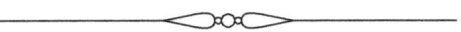

Whenever your life is threatened in some way, such as being in a severe accident that leads to a near-death experience or being given a terminal diagnosis, you tend to reflect on the past with a lot more appreciation for what you have been through.

John and Nathan are my world and were all I could think about in the early days of being diagnosed with CDC. To understand how we became a family, I need to take you back to 1995 and the time John and I were set up by mutual friends.

Meeting my future husband was a whirlwind love affair that swept me up without warning.

I was twenty-nine and working in a factory in Melbourne's south-eastern suburbs. I was a fairly shy person and had struggled with low self-esteem for most of my life. I met Barb when I worked on night shift at the factory. She was a woman who loved to have a chat about things going on in her world, and I loved to listen to her stories. Her humour was engaging and her laugh was infectious. I really enjoyed being around her.

One evening, we had a conversation about how hard it was to find someone compatible to share your life with. A lot of my past boyfriends had not been 'marrying material'. I had just about resigned myself to being single forever, not a bad thing, so I wasn't on the hunt.

Barb's husband, Gary, was a supervisor in another factory not far from where I worked. He was John's supervisor and a friend of many years. The couple had arranged a night out. No pressure, just ten fun people to eat a Chinese meal with and to dance with afterwards. I knew there would be other single people there and I was so nervous. Barb had set me up on a blind date.

> *I had just about resigned myself to being single forever.*

Then I thought how silly I was being. *What have you got to lose?* I said I would go along, but there was an inner voice that kept repeating, *This won't end well*. My track record with relationships so far was not great. I wasn't good at them. Either that or the men I chose weren't good at them. Chances are, it was a combination of the two. I really don't know why it was such an effort to find a compatible partner. I had all but given up. *It's just too hard. Anyway, I'm better off single*. This is what I told myself. I reasoned if things didn't work out and I remained single, I would be able to go on amazing holidays by myself.

I drove around to Barb and Gary's place and left my car there. Barb then picked John up in her car. I sat in the back seat and let him sit in the front. He was skinny and looked like he needed a good feed. His muscly arms caught my attention.

John and I were strategically placed next to each other at the restaurant. At first, we were both a bit shy, but after I consumed a couple of drinks very quickly, I overcame this problem.

> *I really loved his sense of humour.*

With confidence heightened by alcohol, I ended up having a few dances with John. I really loved his sense of humour; he cracked me up laughing. He was probably a lot funnier in the moment, but we had a great time.

When it was time to go home, Barb and Gary insisted we go back to their place and continue the fun night with after-dinner drinks and a game of pool. We parted ways in the early hours of the morning and I was elated that I may have finally found someone who was different, someone who was more compatible with me.

I was expecting a call from John the next day, but it never came. My inner voice was repeating the words, *Here we go again...* and *Why do you bother?* I figured that it was the end. Again.

On the Monday, I received a phone call from John. He was very apologetic that he had not called me on Saturday afternoon when we were meant to arrange to go out. Instead, he had fallen asleep when he arrived home after an early morning stocktaking at his work. He confessed he had fallen asleep and didn't wake up until late Saturday evening. From this point on, I was more cautious because I didn't want to be hurt again.

It didn't take long for me to be swept off my feet by John.

Despite my early uncertainty, it didn't take long for me to be swept off my feet by John. He was unlike any man I had dated before, and about a month later I was totally in love with him. Two months after we met, I moved in with him.

I was impressed with the way he kept his house clean and even put the toilet seat down. I told him jokingly, because of this, I was going to marry him.

In April 1996, we flew to the USA and stayed in Anaheim, Los Angeles, for two weeks. We hired a car, drove to Las Vegas, checked in to Treasure Island and stayed in the penthouse. We

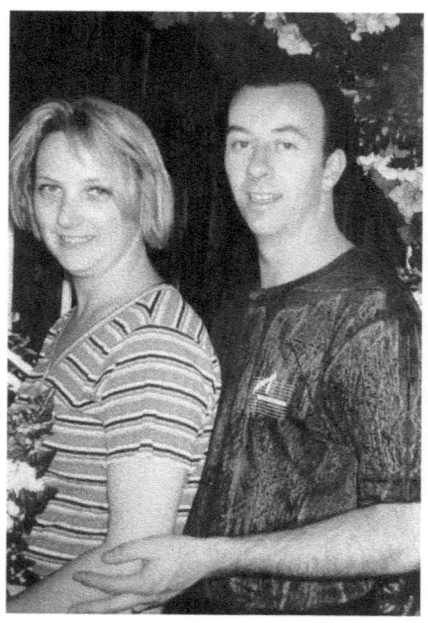

Las Vegas: Chapel by the Courthouse, 1996

were married at the Chapel by the Courthouse on 30 April, only six months after we met.

We didn't talk much in the car on the way back from Las Vegas. When John asked me what I was thinking and why I was so quiet, I confessed that I felt numb and unsure about what we had just done. I felt a little confused about whether it was the right thing to do or not. It turned out, he felt exactly the same. We sat in our mutual uncomfortableness for some time. But John, with his wicked personality, was able to break the tension with one of his silly jokes and the laughter suddenly came back. By the time we reached Anaheim, we were both in good spirits. "What a story we'll have to tell our kids!" John chuckled.

We spent a week in Hawaii before flying home to Melbourne after a total of three weeks away.

I began telling my family of our spontaneous nuptials, bragging about how it only cost me twenty-five dollars to get married. While everyone was surprised, most of the people we told were extremely happy for us. Mixed feelings of "What's the big deal?" and "I'm so glad you didn't get married on my birthday!" came from my siblings.

My family dynamics, like most, have evolved greatly over time.

John and I celebrated our wedding reception party in July 1996 – it remains one of my fondest memories with both of my parents. Both John's family and my side of the family were invited, and lots of our friends. We hired a hot tub and had it

> *My family dynamics, like most, have evolved greatly over time.*

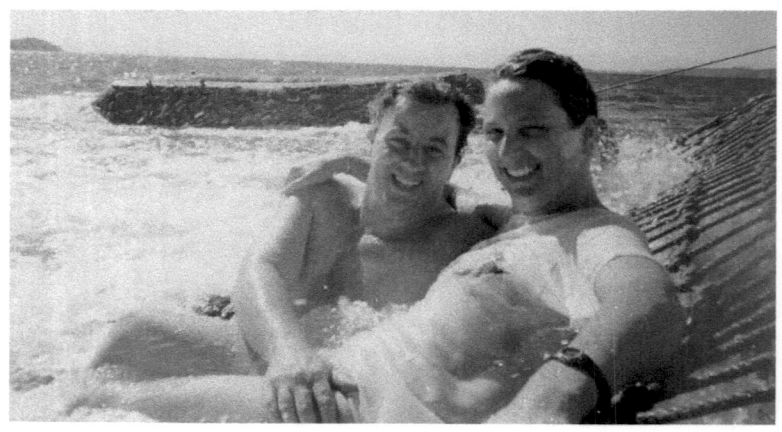

Newlyweds on Great Keppel Island in late 1996

set up in the shed. It became the talking point of our party. My mum and dad came from the country. John's sister Chrissy and his parents came. Only one of my siblings came. The others didn't attend due to 'prior engagements'.

It was a cold night, which was probably why a lot of people didn't turn up. John's crazy friend Nigel decided to jump into the spa in a G-string during the celebrations, which was a highlight of the night.

My mum was always tired and she was most probably in a lot of pain, but I appreciated that she and Dad had gone out of their way to travel that distance for my special night.

It is a night I will always treasure.

I visited Mum as much as I could during her second cancer battle. Sometimes John would come with me and other times he was tied up at work and I went alone.

It was around this time, during a visit to Mum and Dad's, that John and I decided to get a new family pet. John already had Max, a heeler cross, but I felt Max needed company. We bought Flea, a Kelpie cross, from a lady near Heyfield.

When Flea was introduced to Max, we realised Flea was already a little dominating. But over time, Flea didn't bother Max as much and they would play together. Mum took a real shine to Flea and loved to be around her.

Many years later, Max was finding it difficult to walk. The vet had already operated on her a couple of times and told us that, because her stature was the way it was and the fact she was getting on in age now, he thought it not a good idea to do any more operations.

John and I took her home and realised this would most probably be the last night with our beautiful Max. We had her put down the following day and buried her in front of our property.

Flea seemed to be looking for Max for a long time, sniffing around where her bed used to be. This made me think it would be possible now to show Flea lots of affection without sparking the jealousy issue that had become apparent each time I tried to get close to either dog.

Mum deteriorated over three months – in what I now know is palliative care – and I remember the look of annoyance on her face every time she woke up. She

> *I remember the look of annoyance on her face every time she woke up.*

would openly tell me she was upset she was still alive. It was heartbreaking to see her dying this way. I wish I'd been able to do more for her. It hurt so much to see her this way. I wanted to help her but there was only the morphine available at her bedside, supplied automatically through a syringe driver. During her final days, I told a white lie and said I was pregnant. I wanted her to have some hope and something to hold on for... something to brighten her final days.

Mum died on 30 January 1999. She was only sixty-three.

She was the most important influence on my life. I really admire the strength she had. My dad was not the easiest person to get along with and would often stop by the pub on his way home from work. Mum worked night shift and was always there for all of us kids. All while she put on a brave face and endured a long-suffering battle with bowel cancer and then pancreatic cancer. I remember her drawn face towards the end. She was so strong and I miss her terribly.

> *I miss her terribly.*

Mum had been gone for four months when I found out that I was six weeks pregnant. I was a little sad that my mum wouldn't get to meet and know my future child like she knew all her other grandchildren.

Becoming a mum

January 2000

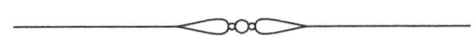

Our healthy son, Nathan, was born on 17 January 2000. I had put on weight and was feeling pretty horrible after Nathan was born. Part of my weight gain was attributed to the fact I had given up smoking. Melbourne weather always seemed to make me catch the seasonal cold and one year it developed into sinusitis and a chest infection. Following a doctor's visit and a chest x-ray, I was told I should quit the cigarettes because I had early signs of emphysema. That was one of the hardest things I've had to do, but after two attempts, an increasing motivation to be fit and healthy in my future, and a desire for Nathan not to be brought up around tobacco smoke and suffer permanent ear damage from second-hand smoke like I had done, I managed to quit the habit after about four months.

Because smoking was no longer in my daily routine, I had replaced the smokes with food. The difficulty with stopping is the habit of having the comfort of the cigarette between the two fingers – it's all a mental test, I know. But this test in my life was one I had to overcome. The food and those extra challenges did not make me happy. And once I realised this, even though I read it everywhere, I had to learn it for myself in my own time. Nathan was a great motivation for my change of ways.

Just before I became pregnant, the company I was working for decided to change from eight-hour shifts to twelve-hour shifts. Although the shifts would be well suited if I didn't have a third person to think about in my future as a new mother, this became a major factor in my decision to accept a redundancy, as I knew it would be impossible for John to work the afternoon shift. There were no options for childcare centres to be open at those times. I left work after eleven years of service.

> *I struggled on and became very depressed.*

Nathan was a challenge when he was a baby. He would sleep for twenty minutes and be awake for twenty minutes. This happened twenty-four hours a day, seven days a week. I was a zombie and suffered undiagnosed postnatal depression. When I went to the maternal health care nurse, she told me I simply had a "snacker and napper" and that was just the way it was going to be. I was at a loss to find a way to get him to eat more so he could sleep longer. Having broken sleep every single night without a chance to catch up by napping during the day was wearing me down. There didn't seem to be a solution. I struggled on and became very depressed.

I cried for help from my doctor, from family members and from John. I felt alone in my battle and hardly anybody gave me good advice. Autism Spectrum Disorder (ASD) was relatively unheard of back then, and I was never advised it was possible that Nathan had this disorder. He went undiagnosed until he was seven years old. That explained the previous seven years of not understanding my demanding child – the sleepless nights, the tantrums and most probably why nobody offered to babysit.

It is now a much more widely known and understood condition. In 2022, the Australian Autism Alliance estimated Australia's autistic population to be around 650,000.[8] ASD is a developmental disorder that affects communication and behaviour. The word 'spectrum' is important because every autistic person is unique.

Autism Spectrum Australia explains that autistic people can display a range of characteristics in their strengths, communication, social interactions, leisure and play.[9] Most of these characteristics become clear in the first two years of life. Nathan had a hypersensitivity to noise and difficulty with social connection and interaction. This was clear when he was often singled out as being naughty and never invited to children's birthday parties.

I felt guilty that Nathan had no interaction with kids his age, nor any siblings as he was an only child. I was excited for him to begin a newly developed program – three-year-old kindergarten. I enrolled him in two sessions a week. I was so hopeful he would develop friendships and be a happier boy. He loved blocks and he'd build towers all day long if you let him. What the kindergarten teachers soon discovered was that if anyone else built a tower, he would just deliberately go over and knock it down. He liked the attention he got when he did it, even though it was negative attention. He was a handful. I was constantly called to come and collect him.

Haircuts were a massive challenge. Nathan's hair was long most of the time when he was young. Nathan could not sit still. When the scissors came towards his head he would thrash around and scream. When he was older, Nathan told me he could *feel* the hair getting cut and it caused him great pain.

Little things became big issues for Nathan. On a trip down to see my dad, Nathan lifted up the glass on the coffee table and dropped it on the floor. It broke and made a mess all over the floor. I cleaned it up, apologised to Dad and said I would replace the glass, which I did. I think it was around this time my dad would refer to Nathan behind my back as 'the little bastard'.

> *I felt I had to justify everything Nathan did.*

I tried to explain Nathan's disability to my family members, even though I knew I wasn't taken seriously. Dad had an attitude that all he needed was a "swift kick up the arse". This seemed to be the perception of other family members as well. I felt I had to justify everything Nathan did: why he did not race up to family members to give them a hug and why he would not want to play with them or look them in the eye. I always felt silent judgement and got the feeling they thought I was making this whole ASD thing up.

Of course, they didn't have to live with it day in, day out. I didn't know how to deal with a child with ASD and it put a lot of strain on my marriage. John was now working afternoon shift, so I was lucky in a way that he didn't see most of it. I don't think he would have been able to cope with Nathan's behaviour. We were lucky our marriage survived. Studies have shown the stress of being a parent to a child with a disability takes a massive toll on families, with an increased risk of divorce compared to couples of children without a disability. For a parent with children with ASD, divorce rates are up to 80%.[10]

There was one occasion when Nathan left his teddy at my sister's house after a visit. I didn't realise until we got home. Given that it was his security item and comforter, he wouldn't be able to sleep without it and I had to go back and get it, which was another forty-minute drive in the dark and wet. Normally, to a child without ASD, it would be okay to collect Teddy in the morning. But not in this case. This was the kind of necessity that became common and what I had to deal with, but my family still believed I was the cause of it all. According to them, I was too soft on Nathan. The only 'support' I received from one of my siblings was a comment that if I didn't discipline Nathan properly by the age of two, he would be unruly and naughty for the rest of his life.

> *John and I love our son unconditionally.*

Nathan had been dubbed a manipulator. His behaviour may appear to be manipulative to the uninformed; I call it his ASD. Nathan has the ability to be able to 'play' people. He has been quite successful in doing this with John. Our son can read his father like a book – I think all kids can to a point. It has caused some tension between us over the years, but John and I love our son unconditionally.

Although my family were judgemental of our family dynamics, I was absolutely devastated when my older sister told me she was going to move to Queensland. I must admit I was a little bit jealous because I had always liked Queensland. Melbourne was too cold, and my best friend, my favourite sister, wasn't going to be here anymore. She was looking for a fresh start. I took comfort in knowing at least I had one other sister still living not far from me.

My sister moved into a unit on the Sunshine Coast and seemed to be settling in very nicely. I missed her terribly, but it didn't seem she was so far away every time we spoke on the phone.

Eating too much through boredom and lack of sleep, I put on a lot of weight. I missed my friends from work and had few social interactions with adults because my hands were tied up with Nathan. I was also upset Nathan would not have his cousins around to grow up with. Just like I never had.

As my weight continued to increase, my energy levels dropped. I was finally able to get employment in a factory when Nathan went to school. But because of my extra weight and the concrete floors, I soon developed sciatica. I was doing all the wrong things. And I soon realised that this pain could become much worse if I didn't act soon.[11] I hated that factory job as most of the people that worked there were men and they weren't very understanding or compassionate. Nathan was in prep and I finished work at the same time he finished school. I had asked my supervisor and management if I could start work five minutes earlier and finish five minutes earlier to ensure I was at the school gate ready to collect Nathan. I told my manager about my situation and how it was highly likely Nathan would run away after school if he wasn't supervised and I wasn't there as soon as he walked through the school gates. The manager stated he was not able to accommodate such a request, as other employees would demand the same 'special' treatment.

Before knock-off time, all the factory workers lined up at the time punch clock. This annoyed me because, even though my workstation was close to the clock, I would be nearly at the end of the queue. By the time I got to punch my card, another five minutes had gone by, and by the time I got into my car and out of the carpark, another five minutes had passed. I was always late collecting Nathan from school. I was singled out if I left my station early. I now realise this was a form of bullying that in this day and age would not be tolerated by HR. But I kept my mouth shut. I had received warnings for doing lots of things the men seemed to get away with. One day I asked one of the men at the start of the line if I could jump into the queue behind him. The men waiting in line erupted in laughter after I mentioned needing to pick my son up from school. "I have to pick up my son," I pleaded. His sarcastic response was, "I have to get to the pub." I resigned the following week!

Nathan had been struggling through the mainstream schooling system. We tried the local school and they quickly found they didn't have the resources to manage him in a full class of students.

We tried another school at Mount Waverley, which boasted having six students to a teacher. They offered cooking classes and special treats when the students behaved and performed well, and they promised us the world for our son, with a 98%

success rate for their students, no matter where they started on the education scale. *This is amazing!* I'd thought as Nathan walked through the school gates. For the first time in a long time, I started to relax.

They promised us the world for our son.

It wasn't long before Nathan told me he was deliberately excluded from a lot of the fun activities because he was branded as the naughty kid. He actually got kicked out of that school, because when the teacher said, "You sit on that mat there, don't move and do your work," he managed to tie his shoelaces into a noose and wrapped them around his neck. He alerted the teacher to it by declaring, "Now you can't make me do my work." He was seven years old at this stage.

He must have been a little shit in class, I don't deny that, but this was a knot the teachers weren't unable to undo straight away. They panicked, especially because knots were somewhat of a speciality for Nathan. Like many ASD kids, he'd fixate on a particular skill or subject matter and devour all of the information he could find on it. Nathan was unharmed, almost triumphant, during this incident. This was his way of being defiant, of telling the teacher that he didn't like what she wanted him to do. I'd witnessed many acts of defiance in my time as his mother, but this particular one earned him an expulsion from the school halfway through the first term. Nathan was obviously in their 2% of unsuccessful children.

I had been trying for a long time to get Nathan into a specialised, government-funded school. I was excited that

Nathan might finally get the help he needed. John was happy to accompany me on a tour of the school, which I won't name here. The tour of the campus was unsettling to say the least. To my horror, I noticed some kids were segregated in enclosures made from pool fencing, like cages, away from the rest of the students. These students were highly intellectually disabled. These children were in much more need of assistance than our son. Nathan's issues seemed so minor when we compared the needs of those children to our own son. Without hesitation, we hightailed it out of there.

Nathan ended up attending five different primary schools. Back then, they didn't have Special Education Units (SEU) in Melbourne, but I was pleasantly surprised to find Queensland did. Queensland Education offered support and inclusion to students with all disabilities.[12] This was another drawcard to the Sunshine State.

> *He managed to tie his shoelaces into a noose and wrapped them around his neck.*

I realised how far behind the schooling options were in Victoria at the time. The SEUs were much better equipped to manage Nathan's needs and keep him engaged in school.

Finding fitness

2008

Having worked in factories for most of my life, the moment came when walking became an effort for me. The sciatic pain was brought on from working in those factories. Standing on a concrete floor all day, and wearing heavy and ill-fitting steel cap boots made for men, had taken a huge toll on me physically. (Women's steel cap boots were not around then). The constant pain and the depression that came with it were my wake-up call.

I knew I needed to lose weight and stop the downward spiral of self-pity. I didn't want to be one of those older people who dies alone on the floor like my aunty had. She'd had a fall and didn't have the strength to get to the phone. It broke my heart. It was also the fuel for the fire in my desire for change – I needed to be there for Nathan.

When I was growing up, my diet wasn't the best. I had no clue about the 'right' food choices. Eating healthily had never been instilled in me. Home Economics was a class at school where we made cakes. I had no clue about nutrients and nowhere to learn. My mum steered away from broccoli and zucchini because she didn't like them. I would eat all of my dinner, even if I didn't like it, just to get dessert.

I confided in one of my sisters one day. I mentioned the sciatica, my general health, and how flat, overweight and depressed I was feeling.

I laughed at the suggestion when she challenged me to enter the Melbourne Marathon ten-kilometre event, which was held at the Melbourne Cricket Ground (MCG). At first, I thought it was a ridiculous idea, but the way I was going, life would not get easier for me. A lot of encouragement from John ignited a new drive in me, and I signed up.

> She challenged me to enter the Melbourne Marathon.

I began my first attempts at a regular running regime, but I found the weight was not shifting easily. I struggled to walk for any sort of distance down the street when I signed up and there were plenty of times I thought, *There is no way on earth I am going to be ready to run ten kilometres in twelve weeks!* A few weeks into it, without the progress I'd hoped to see, I began to have regrets about the commitment I had made.

But one day, my life changed.

It's absolutely true when people say you are not ready to see or hear the things you need to until the moment is just right. I had never noticed the gym next to my workplace at the window furnishing factory before that day, even though I had been walking past it twice a day since I'd started at the factory months earlier.

Now I was aware it was there, it took weeks to get enough courage to walk through the front doors of that gym. I had never set foot in any health and fitness establishment before. In my opinion, only skinny people went into gyms. I walked up to the counter and spoke to the woman wearing tight gym gear and a big fake smile. She was so intimidating to me, even though she was polite, that I couldn't help but judge her in a negative way. I wanted to retreat. But I plucked up the courage to ask her about personal training. Her smile widened and she handed me a business card. I placed it hastily into my bag and left.

It took another couple of weeks before I summoned the courage to dial the number on the card. Danny introduced himself on the phone as I blurted out my intention to become somewhat of a superhero overnight. He sounded lovely and wasn't one to procrastinate – Danny came to my house the following day.

Feeling safe behind the lace curtains in my loungeroom, I watched him walk up the driveway. He had a small frame but walked with a great deal of confidence. I giggled to myself and thought, *How the hell is this guy going to train me?*

Danny measured me, took my blood pressure and talked about my goals. I told him I wanted to run ten kilometres in the event I'd signed up for, which was then only seven weeks away. He had a bit of a friendly giggle, possibly at my naivety, but assured me I would get to my goal. We would start training the next day.

I was so nervous. *What do I wear? What if I can't even make it through a session?* Many thoughts of self-doubt were eating away at me as I watched Danny strut up the driveway the following morning, armed with two-kilo weights and a mat. We spoke about my diet and he told me how I could improve my eating habits. I told him how if I got a little hungry I'd polish off a packet of rice crackers in one sitting. I reasoned, "Because they are rice and rice is good for you, right?" He taught me a lot about diet and exercise. From that point on, I had a feeling of positivity that my life was going to be very different.

> *I had a feeling of positivity that my life was going to be very different.*

Danny trained me for three sessions a week. He only charged $40 an hour and, pretty soon, the weight started falling off as I felt more energetic every day.

I started walking greater distances with Flea, our Kelpie cross. She was great company and very well behaved on a lead. Eventually, Flea and I started running short distances and then did longer runs together. The lean shape of her body allowed her to endure these distances. I built up to running two to three times a week, sometimes with Flea in tow, on top of training three times a week. In later years, Flea and I would run up to ten kilometres together.

My sciatica had gone and for the first time in my life, I felt I could achieve great things. My stress levels were lower and I knew I had found my 'thing'. Running was my meditation; it relieved stress and it got me out of my head and away from a sometimes-turbulent household where the two men in my life often had disagreements. Running was my escape. It was my passion. It boosted my confidence. The only cost of this newly found enjoyment was the price of a new pair of runners to replace my cheap Kmart brand.

The big day arrived – my very first fun run. John and Nathan dropped me off. I was so nervous. I couldn't find my sister in the thousands of people so I ran solo.

I'd done it! I'd set myself a challenge and I'd completed the course.

I was pretty proud of myself for finishing it in one hour and seven minutes. The time wasn't that great in the grand scheme of things, but I'd done it! I'd set myself a challenge and I'd completed the course. I felt on top of the world and for the first time in a long time, I felt physically fit and confident.

I continued running. Sometimes on a Sunday morning, I would run sixteen kilometres or further. I entered 'Run for the Kids', which is a sixteen-kilometre run through the city of Melbourne. I kept training with Danny, losing weight and getting stronger. Danny let loose with another laugh when I told him my intention to do the twenty-three-kilometre Apollo Bay Half Marathon in another two months. I confess I was now addicted to fitness.

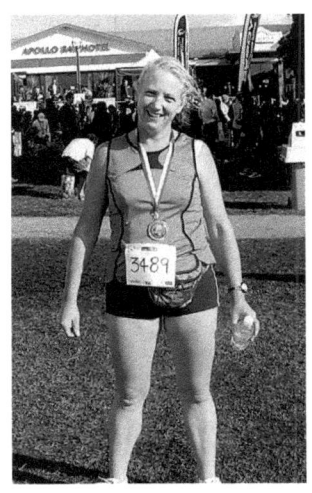

Apollo Bay Half Marathon in 2008

The big move

July 2009

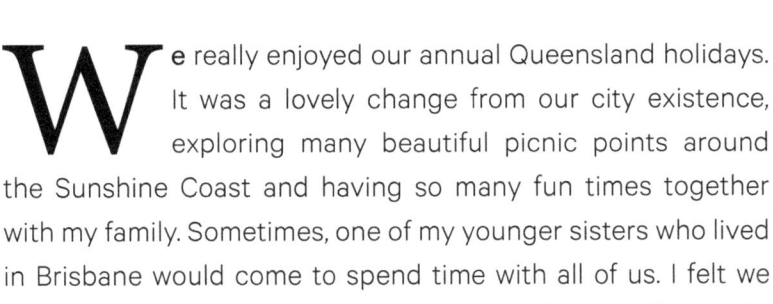

We really enjoyed our annual Queensland holidays. It was a lovely change from our city existence, exploring many beautiful picnic points around the Sunshine Coast and having so many fun times together with my family. Sometimes, one of my younger sisters who lived in Brisbane would come to spend time with all of us. I felt we were starting to reconnect and heal our old wounds. At the end of every holiday, when it was time to say goodbye, I always cried, because I knew I wouldn't see my closest sister who lived on the Sunshine Coast for another year.

My mum used to have a saying: "Melbourne may be a big city, but it can be the loneliest place in the world." John was working afternoon shift and I was isolated with Nathan. I now saw quite clearly what Mum was talking about.

John realised how much I was missing my sisters, and after many discussions about a better life, I managed to convince him to move north. I was excited. Now Nathan could get to know his cousins. I felt a little bit sad John's sister and mother wouldn't see Nathan as much, but I reasoned it was for the best. John's sister Chrissy had many friends in her life, whereas we didn't. We packed up everything and moved to the Sunshine Coast.

John, Nathan, Flea and I had been packing a shipping container for months in preparation for our big move. We had a trailer with John's VW car shell packed tight on it – it was a work in progress. We decided to travel on the inland roads. Just out of Melbourne on the busy freeway, the wind ripped the tarp off the car on the trailer, forcing us to pull over and resecure it in a fluster. We were hoping this wouldn't be a sign of things to come. Luckily, things got better, and Flea was coping quite well with travelling. I really didn't like the idea of her being in a cage on a plane, so she came with us in the car. We booked accommodation that allowed pets in the rooms. It was fantastic that Flea could be with us the whole time. She would lie on

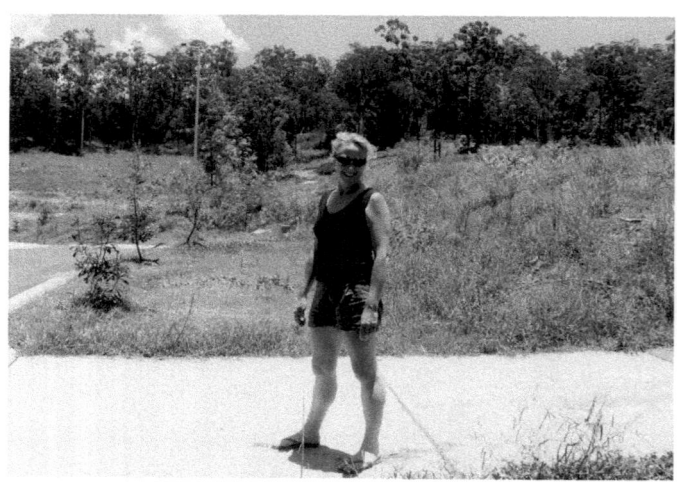

Assessing our 'blank canvas' which would later become our home – Mooloolah Valley 2009

The big move

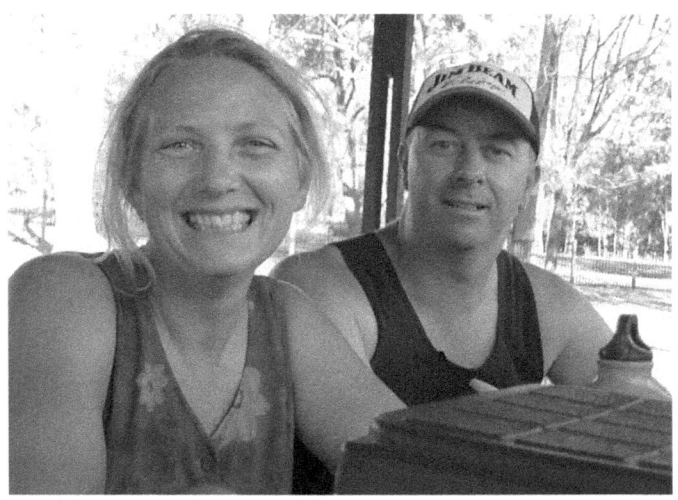

Excited for our new life on the Sunshine Coast

the back seat with her head on my lap. Nathan, being around 170cm tall, sat in the front, while John drove most of the way. Flea was able to 'tell' me when she needed a wee stop. We split the journey into three legs and arrived on the Sunshine Coast in July 2009.

Before we moved, John was able to secure a job in Caloundra. We had organised for a shed to be built on a block of land in the hinterland town of Mooloolah Valley before we left Victoria. When we arrived on the Coast, only the outer walls had been completed. There was no running water or electricity at this stage. We dropped off the trailer at the shed and stayed at my sister's house for two weeks while we got the necessary utilities connected. For six months we had to make do with a portable loo, which I emptied every day. We showered in a solar camping shower we hung up outside in the sun. We roughed it like this for about twelve months. Over time, we were able to build internal walls in the shed, install a flushing toilet in the bathroom, and fit a reverse cycle air-conditioner to make it as comfortable as possible, especially for Nathan who didn't need extra heat to make him 'melt down'. Things were looking up. Every second or third weekend we had picnics and barbecues together with my siblings.

The first fractures started to appear in my relationship with my sisters after about eighteen months. I had no idea what changed their views on our friendship. I had no control over what was happening but soon learned that my new friends held a valuable place in my heart.

> The first fractures started to appear in my relationship with my sisters.

I continued my healthy ways and participated in the Caloundra Foreshore Fun Run, which was an annual major fundraiser. I also began my annual entry into the Sunshine Coast Cross Country Series and the Sunshine Coast Trail Run Festival.

Through exercise and my learned love for running, I felt more empowered to deal with the challenges that would pop up in my life. I looked after myself well during that period of my life. I was becoming fit and healthy. I felt so strong and looked forward to my morning runs, where I could solve a lot of problems while listening to the rhythmic fall of my feet on the footpath. I felt inspired to help others and my healthy ways built my confidence and self-esteem.

The big move

Without a doubt, I knew Danny had changed my life. I was so impressed with what my personal trainer had done for me, I decided to become a personal trainer too. I completed a Diploma of Fitness and emerged fresh from my course with visions of transforming people's lives through fitness. I was so confident this would work.

However, once I finished my diploma in 2011, I found it hard to get clients, even though I charged only $40 an hour while others were charging more than double that. I found the advertising cost too much, and where we lived on the Sunshine Coast, there was too much competition in the fitness industry. I felt I didn't stand a chance. I wasn't the usual young gym junkie that appeared on the cover of *Runner's World* magazine.

I decided to hold group fitness classes at a new local park, which was opening to the public a few weeks later. John and I purchased gym equipment from a studio that was closing down and stored it all in the garage. Once the house was built, my intention was to have a studio where I could train people from home, which would help me out with the juggle of being a mum and running a business.

One of the major expenses we had when we first moved was our intention to build an in-ground pool. One of my neighbours saw the swimming pool propped up on its side on the nature strip across the road in preparation for being put into the ground the following week. She knocked on my door and asked me if I would hold aqua aerobics classes. Although I had no training in this field, I studied quickly to upskill and ran classes in our swimming pool once it was installed. I had four ladies come at one stage and they all seemed to enjoy it immensely, so the classes continued for some time. I focused on making my group fitness classes in the park a success, and at the park's open day in July 2011, I walked around handing out fliers to spread the word.

I was excited that the response seemed quite positive. I made an A-frame sign and had it on the side of the road near the park so people driving past would know about my group fitness sessions.

While running my aqua and circuit classes, I was trying to cope with living in the garage and finding a suitable school for Nathan, as the first state school we'd tried since moving to the Sunshine Coast didn't have the capacity to cater for his needs. I continued working part-time in a curtain-making shop to have some income coming in while I attempted to establish my personal training business. I suggested my niece and sister come and join in one of my training sessions, but my sister rolled her eyes at my suggestion. As far as she was concerned, it was all a waste of time and a big waste of money.

Most trainers were young and did not have the same commitments as I did. My responsibility as a mum meant the only time I could run fitness classes was at 7am on Saturday mornings. One of the ladies who joined the class was very friendly and boosted my confidence. She must have seen how terrified I was because I was never one to be in charge. I was the kid who wet her pants at 'show and tell' in school. She was a great motivator. She was so understanding and supportive. She made it easy for me to run the class and understood my anxiety and my dry sense of humour. Other people came and went over the years, but the group had four regulars who would become my friends.

I held the sessions regardless of the weather. The only time I didn't was when I was sick with a cold. We all formed a bond. Occasionally we would hold the sessions at different locations and enter different challenges throughout the year. One year, we went to Tamborine Mountain, west of the Gold Coast, to complete a vertical challenge. We all had a wonderful time and motivated each other throughout the tough course.

While I was building a group of lovely friends through my fitness classes, I was beginning to feel more and more on the outer within my own family.

The circuit ladies and I would all vent to each other about things that were going on in our lives and found that this was good, not only for our physical health but for our mental health as well. We were very helpful to each other on our down days too. When we trained away from the park, we would sometimes go for breakfast afterwards.

When I was first employed by the curtain shop on the Sunshine Coast, I told my employer of Nathan's learning difficulties and said sometimes the school would ring me and I would need to go and collect him. I was upfront about how I couldn't be reliable and work longer hours and they were accepting of this at first.

> *My employer hired another worker to replace me.*

However, while I was away on holiday, my employer hired another worker to replace me. I didn't find out until my return. There was a new face and when I asked the other woman what her role was, I realised she was doing my job. I was told they would find something else for me to do. I was then given jobs like dusting and cleaning the showroom and toilets. I knew in my heart they were trying to drive me out of my job, and I was very upset with this new situation. Although I had my Saturday circuit and the aqua classes bringing in some money, I knew being a trainer in fitness was not going to be sustainable if I were to leave the safety of employment to run my own business full-time. I was waiting for some lightbulb to go off in my head that would guide me to the solution.

It was late in 2012, on my way home from what I knew would be my final day at work at the curtain shop – I'd finally had enough – when I heard an advertisement on the radio spruiking a nursing course.

The Sunshine Coast was in the midst of having its brand-new hospital built and there was going to be a huge demand for new staff, so I thought about becoming a nurse. I already had a liking for human anatomy and health. The thought of a more steady and reliable income was also a great drawcard, and John was on board, as he could see how I lit up when I spoke to him about becoming a nurse. **This was my aha moment!** As soon as I got home, I took my leap of faith and rang the number to enrol.

I was ready to try to make a difference in people's lives. My mother was a nurse, and even though she had encouraged me many years ago to choose a nursing career, I didn't have the passion back then. I credit Nathan with giving me the gift of patience. He kept me grounded and gave my life a purpose. I knew that, because of these skills, I would be a good nurse. My mum would have been so proud.

The course ran for eighteen months and during this time, we were still chipping away at building a house, John was hating his job and Nathan was hating school. I, on the other hand, was loving life. I was studying, teaching aqua aerobics, holding circuit every Saturday morning, and being a mum. I especially loved it when my sister would come over and have a coffee and share her delicious homemade cakes with me. We'd make small talk and laugh about silly things. But I felt I had to be wary with some things I spoke about to her, as she would make it known she was uncomfortable and often disagreed with my opinion. I still loved my family unconditionally however... because that's what families do.

That same year my siblings had arranged to meet at a park north of Brisbane to celebrate Christmas. We were to be there at 11am. Unfamiliar roads led us to being lost and we were fifteen minutes late. After giving apprehensive hugs all round, we started unloading the car and getting things ready for the barbecue. We were quite surprised to see everyone else was finishing off their food and beginning to pack up. John and I looked at each other and couldn't believe what we were seeing. Half an hour later, my younger sister announced she would be leaving with her partner and son as they had somewhere else to go. Then my other sister left with her partner. Soon John, Nathan and I finished our lunch on our own. We couldn't understand why they invited us to a place almost an hour away to spend just half an hour with us. John and I couldn't understand why both my sisters were being so nasty. I am still no wiser.

I was enjoying my nursing course and was making lots of friends. I couldn't wait to get out in the field and put my new skills into practice. I continued to train, run and keep fit, as well as study. I found that while I ran, I could solve a lot of nursing problems in the assignments I had to complete. The solutions seemed to drop right out of the sky and into my mind, which further strengthened my love for this practice.

> *I couldn't wait to get out in the field and put my new skills into practice.*

The Diploma of Fitness study had helped me understand the human body even more. I met some lovely friends and enjoyed the fact that I was not the oldest student in the nursing class. After I graduated in March 2013, I was so excited. I felt comforted knowing my mum would be happy with my new career choice. That feeling of finally having a meaningful job and a fulfilling career was the best I had ever felt.

I was finally qualified and able to do something with my life and I would never have to work in a factory again.

Our class held a graduation dinner at a little restaurant in town, where we took photos of each other wearing the one and only mortarboard cap. It was such a fun night but a sad one as well as I knew I wouldn't see most of my new friends again. However, at the same time I knew that once I was in the workforce, I would make new friends. I saw this as just one door closing for another one to open.

I threw myself into finding work. I was surprised how quickly I was offered a job. It was a pleasant surprise after the uphill

The big move

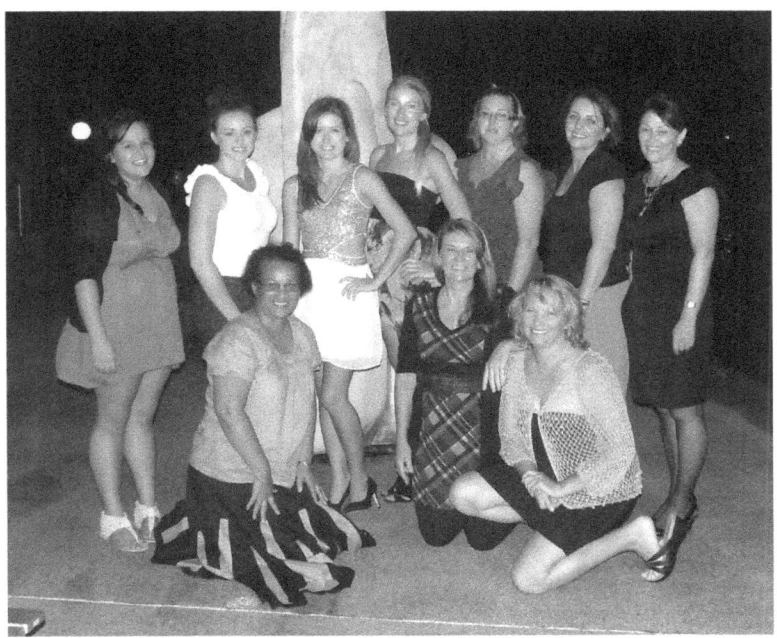

Class of 2013 – Diploma of Nursing graduation. I'm in the front row on the right

battle I'd had as a personal trainer. At one stage, I was working two casual jobs and one on-call job, all in aged care. The work involved visiting people in their homes and assisting them to get ready for the day. Although there wasn't a lot of nursing involved, I enjoyed it just the same and I knew it would provide the necessary experience.

Our own house was nearly finished and soon we would be able to move in. I was pretty fed up with living in the shed. It always felt dusty and dirty because of the unsealed concrete floor. There was no room for the three of us to get away from each other. It felt like cabin fever – we were always standing on each other's toes.

I phoned Dad one day to see how he was going and to see if he had recovered from the flu that seemed to be staying with him. He revealed he had just got out of hospital for problems with his prostate. He'd kept this all under the radar and I really had no idea this was what he was going through. The doctors couldn't do much for him because of his age and because of his health. He thought it funny when the medical team had to put his bed near the nurse's station because he had continued to smoke in his hospital room. The nurses needed to keep an eye on him so he didn't keep flouting the strict no-smoking policy. He was sent home after about a week and never really got back to being himself again.

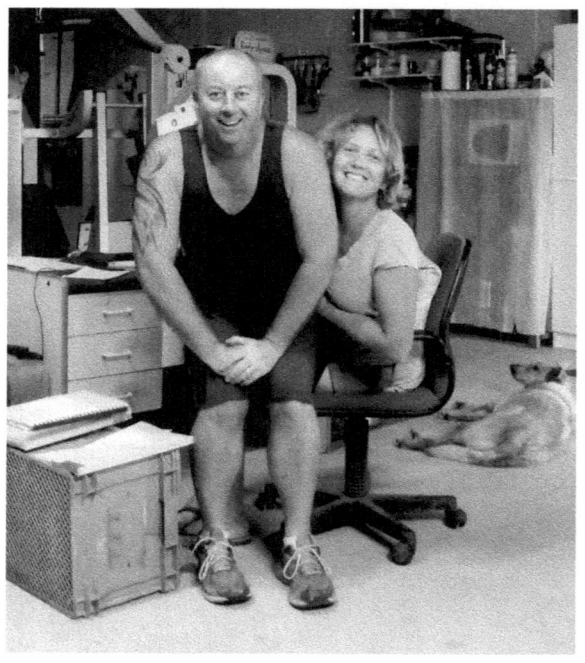

Living in the shed wasn't always fun

The big move

When I wasn't at work, I was busy tiling and painting the house, mothering, and pounding the pavement on my runs. Saturday's fitness class had become more of a social outlet for the girls, as they seemed to oppose hard physical exercise and protested if I tried to get them out of their comfort zones. I knew Dad was still unwell, but with his upbringing, where he learned not to worry others with his own issues, he told me it was nothing major and "nothing for me to worry about." And, of course, I believed there was nothing for me to be overly concerned about.

The symptoms

July 2013

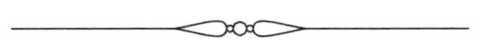

Every Sunday, I got up, dressed in my running gear, filled my water bottle and headed out the door. John and Nathan were still sound asleep in bed as I closed the door gently behind me. Instead of running my usual route around home, I was preparing for my fourth Caloundra Foreshore Fun Run and I had a mission to beat my personal best time and complete the ten-kilometre course in under one hour.

After one of these training runs, I went to the toilet and noticed an off-colour in the toilet bowl. *Nathan didn't flush again!* I flushed the toilet while muttering things about filthy teenagers and hopped into the shower. I went to the toilet again later in the morning, but this time, I noticed a bright red stream in my urine.

I wasn't completely shocked. I'd experienced a similar thing before when I'd been diagnosed with a urinary tract infection. I made an appointment with the doctor as soon as I could. I was always vigilant with my health, and completing my nursing diploma had cemented this even more. *It's better for them to tell me it's just a UTI than for me to miss something major.*

I kept watch every time I went to the toilet in the lead-up to my appointment and didn't see blood again for a few days. The doctor said it was most probably an infection and prescribed a course of antibiotics. I found some leftover urinalysis test strips from my nursing studies and decided I'd conduct my own urine test. I didn't really understand why I was taking the antibiotics because my temperature was normal and I didn't have any of the usual symptoms of a urinary tract infection.

The gut feeling that something wasn't adding up wouldn't go away, so I made another appointment about one week later to see a different doctor. I was really surprised at the thoroughness of this new doctor. He asked me an abundance of questions and referred me immediately for an ultrasound examination.

The following day, I received a call from the doctor: the type of call I never thought I would receive in my life.

I was informed they had found a tumour on my kidney.

I was informed they had found a tumour on my kidney. The type of tumour could not be identified, but the doctor advised there was a possibility it could be cancerous. I felt sick. *The word cancer relates to other people, not me!* I was in utter disbelief.

I was trying so hard not to shake as I shared the results with John as soon as I got home. He was a calming influence on me and cautioned me not to worry too much, as nothing was confirmed. I also rang my sister and then the tears came

The symptoms

flooding out of me. She was never one to be openly emotional and said she couldn't understand why I was losing it. She made a comment about me being a hypochondriac and self-centred and then reprimanded me. She then directed her anger at the doctor, who she said should not have told me about the possibility of the tumour being cancerous at this early stage.

As I was driving to another doctor's appointment I felt I should let Dad know what was going on with my health, to keep him in the loop. I told him my news and he seemed to be in disbelief. He reassured me everything would be okay. I told him I was nervous and asked him how his health was. But as usual, he replied, "Not bad." I took his word for it. But my sister called me later that evening and scolded me. She was disgusted that I had called him. Apparently, he was worse than he was letting on and was struggling with his own poor health. As far as she was concerned, I should not be bothering him with my health issue as he had his own.

I was booked in two days later to have a CT scan. The wait for the results of the scan seemed to take forever. I tried so hard not to let it sit in my mind. Waiting is not something I am great at. I was unable to vacate the anxiety. This is now what I know as 'scanxiety'.[13] This would be a part of my new life. It's the anxiety that comes with waiting for the results of a scan. When my doctor finally rang, it was with the sentence you never want to hear: "I need you to come and see me right away."

The receptionist booked me in that day and I didn't have to spend very long in the waiting room for the hammer to fall. The doctor broke the news. The tumour was 7cm long. Although the presence of cancer was still unconfirmed, I was listed as a category two patient, which meant the wait for an operation could be up to three months. They would go in and remove my kidney with the hope of getting all of the tumour out at the same time. They could then send off a segment of the tumour to see what it was they were dealing with.

While I waited for my surgery date to be locked in, life was pretty well normal on a surface level. The girls from circuit training were very supportive and completely shocked when I told them what had unfolded.

> How could he have gone from "not bad" to knocking on death's door?

My sister told me she was taking time off from her casual position to go and help Dad out by cutting firewood and helping him around the acreage in country Victoria. I didn't think much about it. I wanted to accompany her as I hadn't seen Dad for a while, but I had to think of myself and Nathan, who never coped well without me around. And John wouldn't have been able to cope well with Nathan's likely tantrums.

It wasn't until late July I was told that, if I wanted to see Dad for the last time, I would have to come and see him very soon. *How could he have gone from "not bad" to knocking on death's door?* My sisters had mentioned Dad wasn't well previously but never really told me how dire the situation was.

I was completely taken aback by this news. Dad had always glossed over his health when we spoke, most likely to shield me from worrying about him, but now I realised the full force of

The symptoms

what he was up against – prostate and lung cancer – and it was a complete shock.

Once I had the realisation that Dad was going to die, I had to make a quick decision. After a two-month wait, my surgery was booked in and I'd just completed all of the preadmission paperwork. I was concerned with my own health. I didn't like the idea of being so far away from the hospital where my records were kept and my history known. I was passing blood every time I went to the toilet at this stage. I had visions of fainting from the blood loss. John and I discussed all the pros and cons and decided it would be best to take the risk of travelling if it meant I could see Dad alive and say my goodbyes. But it would most likely mean I would not be able to go to his funeral.

I booked a shuttle bus from the Sunshine Coast to take me to the airport in Brisbane early on a Wednesday morning. I then caught a plane to Melbourne at 8am and hopped on a train to Gippsland, Victoria. The train stopped twenty minutes from where my dad lived. After about an hour of negotiations with the car hire place, I eventually hired a car and drove out to Dad's house.

When I arrived, my sister rushed out to greet me. She spoke in a hushed tone as she told me Dad was resting on the couch in the lounge room. I followed her back into the house and couldn't believe what I saw. He looked so ill. With his eyes closed, his face was drawn and sunken. It is a vision of him that will never leave my mind. The only way I could see that this man was in fact my father was through his eyes when he finally managed to

> *His face was drawn and sunken.*

open them. I felt a wave of emotion overcome me, but I withheld my tears. I did not want Dad to see how sad I was.

I stood there watching him, trying to make sense of everything that was happening. It was extremely hard to make out that the person lying on the couch was the same person I had known all of my life and who I had spoken to on the phone the previous week.

Dad lived on a self-sufficient acreage. The pumps had to be tended to daily for water. The solar electricity batteries needed to be checked. Something he easily did when he was much fitter. I was relieved my sister was able to assist as much as she could. She felt unable to leave Dad to tend to the pumps, which meant she couldn't shower at the house. She had to go into town to the local pool. She was relieved I was there to take watch over Dad's care while she went into town for a shower. In the time she was gone, I knelt at my father's side and told him how much I loved him. He was dosed up on morphine, but in his lucid moments, when his eyes fixed on me and softened, he told me he loved me too and reassured me. We only had small windows of time before the pain relief drugs took hold again and he drifted off to sleep. Even in this painful time, he was still concerned about my wellbeing and making me feel safe.

I was sitting at the kitchen table talking quietly with my sister. I told her how frightened I was, so far away from the hospital in the condition I was in. I'd decided I would only stay one night and would leave the next day.

I had to switch back to my own reality. All I could see was the toilet bowl turning crimson every time I went. I was dizzy, tired and so far away from help if an emergency arose.

The symptoms

The following morning, I said goodbye to Dad and told him I loved him. He'd chosen to stay on the couch as he didn't like to be in his own bed. It was here that he spent the remaining days of his life. I gave my sister a hug and left the house. I knew his death was imminent. There was a heavy weight on my heart, knowing this would be the last time I would see my father.

The trip back home was a long one and I was exhausted when I walked through the door of my own home that evening. The following day, I talked to John about my visit. At 11pm that night, my sister rang to tell me Dad had just died.

The funeral was organised on the same day my surgery had been scheduled. I reasoned that I had seen my dad alive, and I knew he would understand my decision. The choice was the right one. I was happy I was able to see my father one last time.

> *This would be the last time I would see my father.*

I knew my dad would not want me to mess with my health, and the logistics of changing a surgery date through the public health system were crazy. There was a possibility I would be put back at the end of the list and have to restart the three-month waiting period. As we still didn't know if this tumour was sinister, it was a chance I was unwilling to take. I was relieved that at least I had been able to spend those twenty-four hours by his side.

The treatment

August 2013

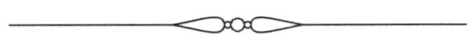

This is where you joined me at the start of the book. It's just a few days after my rare cancer diagnosis. I had survived the surgery, knew what I was up against, and I was determined to win my battle with collecting duct carcinoma.

I remained positive at my preliminary appointment, where they discussed what was going to happen and introduced me to the staff on duty at the hospital. I made light of what was going on to the nurse and John. This was the way I dealt with things. Without humour, I didn't know how I was going to make it through.

On the inside, I was anxious and worried. My body was going to be poisoned. Chemotherapy was all new to me. Even though both my parents had different types of cancer, my mum didn't have the choice of chemotherapy as it wasn't available at the time. She later succumbed to the secondaries of bowel cancer. It would most likely have been

My body was going to be poisoned.

refused by my dad if it were offered. If detected early and treated, the Cancer Council says the five-year survival rate for prostate cancer is 95%.[14] However, being an old-school, manly man, my father never sought medical advice. Then it was too late. He had smoked cigarettes for most of his life and it is common knowledge that this is the main cause of lung cancer.

For the uninitiated, chemotherapy is the use of drugs to destroy cancer cells. The primary aim of chemotherapy is to stop the cancer cells from growing, dividing and spreading, although it can also affect healthy cells in its quest to slow or eliminate cancer.[15] Doctors use this method because cancer cells usually reproduce much faster than healthy cells and therefore the chemotherapy will impact more of them.

In my case, the oncologist wanted to destroy any cancer cells that may be lingering following the removal of my kidney and the tumour. 'To mop up' were the words he used to describe the drugs' purpose. There was a possibility some cancer cells had made their way into my bloodstream and lymph nodes. There was a high likelihood they were circulating around waiting to pop up in another organ. When this happens, it's called metastatic cancer.[16]

I did not hesitate, with the possibility of metastasis occurring, and was totally ready to kill the bastards.

Treatment is usually determined by the type of cancer you have and how large the tumour may be. The general health of a person will determine the dosage. I was the healthiest I had ever been and young enough. I was positive I would be able to cope with the myriad side effects I might come up against.

The treatment

The only side effects from chemotherapy I had heard about were hair loss and vomiting. I was most probably advised of them all, but these were the only ones I could recall. The Cancer Council lists the following as possible chemotherapy side effects, most of which are temporary and can be treated or managed if they arise:[17]

- Nausea and vomiting
- Diarrhoea or constipation (often due to anti-nausea medication)
- Fatigue
- Anaemia
- Mouth sores or ulcers
- Increased risk of infection
- Increased risk of bruising
- Hair loss
- Muscle weakness
- Skin sensitivity to sunlight (specific drugs only)
- Changes to the nails
- Dry or tired eyes
- Changes in appetite
- Changes in fertility
- Thinking and memory changes.

What was not on their list was:

- Early onset menopause/chemotherapy-induced menopause.[18]

There was no mention on the website of medical cannabis as a complementary or alternative therapy. The oncologist told John and me that there was little information available about the course of action to take for the type of cancer I had and they were going to treat me as if I had bladder cancer. I felt confident that whatever chemical cocktail they injected would eliminate any cancer cells that might be lurking in my bloodstream. He was a specialist. He knew best. Being a mentally strong person, I told the doctor this whole chemotherapy thing would be a walk in the park. I intended to maintain my usual exercise regime, which included taking my beloved Flea around the block every day and running two to three times a week.

In October 2013, I went into the hospital for the first chemotherapy treatment, carrying an overnight bag. My nerves were completely frazzled as the unknown loomed large in my mind. This overnight practice became commonplace for the first day of all of my chemo cycles. They wanted to monitor me to ensure my remaining kidney would be able to handle the toxicity of the drugs.

It was an awful feeling walking past the maternity ward, looking at the happy couples sharing the joy of their newborns and new life. Their smiling faces made me feel quite sick at the thought of my looming death. I wondered if anybody else felt like me. Surely, they could have put the wards at opposite ends of the hospital.

I sat in a chair in the oncology department, waiting to be called. I then went into the chemotherapy ward. This is when it hit me. *This is real.* I was shocked to see so many sick people looking fatigued. *Surely, I am not that sick? Nor am I as old as these people*. It just didn't seem fair. I was given two chemotherapy drugs: Gemcitabine[19] and Cisplatin[20] – common bladder cancer drugs – through a cannula on the back of my hand. The drugs were the strongest they could give and my body initially dealt with them quite well.

Despite my uncertainty about how the treatment would affect me, I remained positive the chemotherapy would kill the cancer and life would continue as normal. The needle went into the back of my hand quite easily and for the next four hours, I ate sandwiches and had a cup of tea and watched a couple of movies. I drank three litres of water prior to and during the treatment. This became a regular practice after the doctors informed me, if I didn't look after my remaining kidney, there would be a possibility I would have to go on dialysis. My mission was to ensure I flushed the chemicals out of my body as fast as I could.

The next morning, after a horrible night of not sleeping very well in the hospital environment, John came to pick me up. I was trying to be my chirpy self, but I was so exhausted. I felt okay for two days after the big dose of chemotherapy, continuing to walk around the block with Flea and trying my utmost to continue with life.

The third day was a completely different story. It hit me with full force. I had a headache and felt like vomiting all day. It felt like the worst hangover I had ever endured and nothing I could do would help it go away. I spent most of the time curled up on the couch because I could hardly walk. The medication they gave me stopped me from vomiting, but it didn't take away the horrible feeling of wanting to vomit. This feeling lasted for another week and was with me both day and night. All I could do was try to drink lots of water and continue to eat so I could keep up my strength.

On week two of the chemotherapy, only Gemcitabine was given. I was relieved I didn't have to stay in hospital overnight and could come home afterwards. I began to find it very hard to walk around the block every day. *My energy levels were the worst they had ever been.* But each week, towards the end of the cycle, I would start to feel better. Week four was a recovery period and I didn't have any drugs. This was cycle one complete. There were three more just like it to go.

During the second cycle, my body felt weaker still. I could only make it halfway around the block with Flea. I felt really ill driving to the hospital, which was perched on the side of a steep hill. I was struggling physically but they don't issue disability parking stickers for chemotherapy patients, so I had to endure the added torment of arriving with enough time to find a car park, which added to the stress. I then had the ordeal of trudging up the hill in the humid Queensland summer with sweat pouring from my forehead.

John invited my family over for an afternoon barbeque to lift my spirits during one of my cycles. After talking and laughing while we ate, I decided it would be a suitable time to talk about important matters. However, the barbeque was cut short when I asked to speak about my mortality and future funeral plans. The conversation upset my niece when I spoke about my request to be cremated. She said it made her feel uncomfortable. I was accused of trying to take the conversation away from being about Dad to focus on myself. But I felt it had to be discussed as soon as possible as I was seeing my family less often.

Walking Flea around the block became an almost impossible mission. After two months of chemotherapy, I could no longer make it to the top of the steps at my house or more than five minutes from home on what were once my daily walks. My body was swollen and puffy. My eyes were almost closed. My breath was becoming laboured and my body was tired.

> *I asked to speak about my mortality and future funeral plans.*

I felt upset when, on two occasions when I was to stay in hospital overnight, I showed up for treatment only to find there were no available beds and my meal was not on the list, so sandwiches were my dinner. I felt like I was invisible. I wondered if the staff chatting away and wandering the hallways actually tried to sleep in one of the rooms. I could not understand why they spoke and giggled so loud. But then, I am a light sleeper. The bed was so small compared to my bed at home. It made a lot of noise every time I rolled over. I reasoned with myself that all I had to do was put up with it for one night each month. In my drained state, it was hard to maintain my original positivity – that I would make it through this.

On Christmas Eve 2013, I was able to come home after spending the night in hospital. It was a quiet Christmas. Nathan and John looked after me as best they could. Not only was I dealing with the physical effects of the chemotherapy, I was also struggling to understand why my own family had turned their backs on me. The emotional fallout of this was intense.

At the start of the third month of chemotherapy cycle, it took four attempts to find my vein to insert the canula. When it wouldn't go into the vein and went under the skin instead, the "slight scratch" the nurse stated I would feel was a burning sensation that wouldn't stop and the back of my hand swelled up. It was so painful. I could feel my body tense up. It was as if my body was trying to hide my veins in an attempt to stop the constant needles from coming. The lumps under my skin in these areas are permanent reminders of the chemotherapy process. Whenever I become conscious of them, my mind is always transported back to this particular treatment and the intense feelings that came with it.

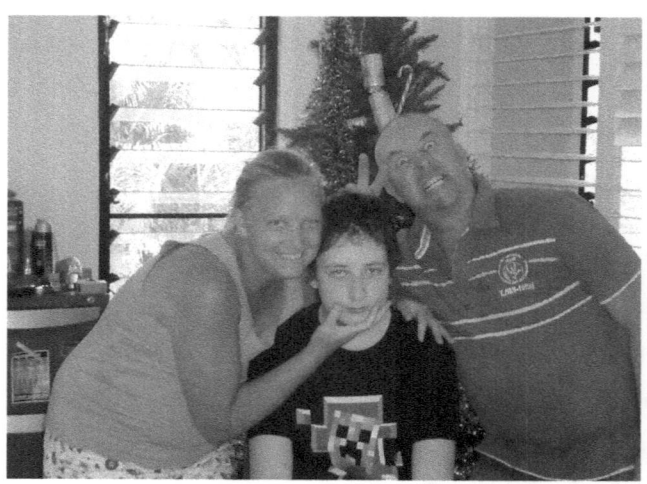

Christmas 2013

The treatment

I was given a card that told staff at the hospital I was a chemotherapy patient. I was warned that if I had a temperature I was to come in straight away as I could have an infection. I used this card for the first time during the third cycle when I developed cellulitis, which is a bacterial skin infection that can become life-threatening if not treated quickly.[21] It was 11pm and my temperature was 39 degrees. I took paracetamol and put cold washes on my forehead. But my temperature wasn't dropping. I couldn't believe the dirty looks I got from patients in the emergency ward when I produced my 'gold' card at reception and was immediately whisked away to a room. To them, I had jumped the queue. I spent three days in hospital hooked up to intravenous antibiotics to be treated and recover from this infection in my hand and lower arm.

By the end of the four months, my body had endured enough. My veins were retreating from being constantly poked and prodded. I was physically and mentally spent. Summer had arrived with the full force of a traditional sweltering Queensland season and I started spending hours in the pool, sweating, crying and trying to be as active as possible no matter how much my body protested. The water hid my tears and after long sessions in there, I had to get out, as my fingers were getting very crinkly from being in the pool too long.

The water hid my tears.

People were surprised at how good I looked while I underwent treatment. They had no idea I felt like death on the inside. Some would comment on how I still had most of my hair. I felt like losing my hair would be a small price to pay if I were to live. Some even suggested that perhaps my chemotherapy dosage wasn't strong enough as I hadn't had that stereotypical side effect.

While I was on chemotherapy, I tried my best to continue with my group fitness classes. I sat in the car on my worst days and instructed the girls which exercises to carry on with. They obliged, and these mornings were a welcome distraction to the unrest I felt within my body and mind whenever I had time to pause.

"The cancer may be rare and aggressive, but you are even more rare and aggressive," one of the girls said. I really appreciated how she lifted my spirits. I sat in the car with a towel on my lap, being prepared to vomit while the group did the walk or whatever other activity I had arranged for them. I didn't feel like I was a very good role model as I was pretty much incapacitated. The thought of doing anything would make me dry retch.

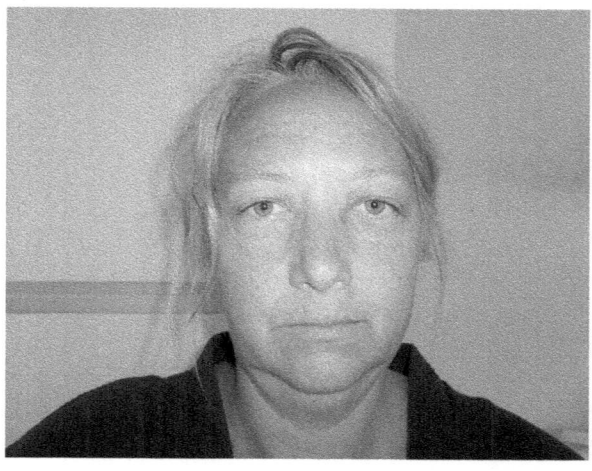

January 2014 – halfway through chemo

Sometimes, if I had enough energy, I walked with them, and I loved the spark this brought to me. The feeling of being physically fit was something I craved, as I was aware my fitness was in a fast decline. The ladies were so sympathetic and understanding, and I asked John if he could run the class when I was at my worst. He was happy to help where he could and the ladies embraced him openly. They supported me without question through this time and it gave me strength to carry on.

There were many nights while I was undergoing chemotherapy when I would have horrible dreams and feel myself falling. I'd wake up with a start to find sweat dripping off my body. Every time I closed my eyes at night – or in the early hours of the morning if sleep was escaping me – I would have a niggling thought: *Am I going to wake up?* Perhaps waking up shaking was linked with this mindset. I'll never know, but there was definitely a lot of anxiety.

The feeling of being physically fit was something I craved.

Sometimes I wrote poetry at silly times. It was a way to fend off the tears that threatened to come whenever I had time to think. It usually happened when I needed sleep.

Nathan's poem

Some may worry about things,
Like how they are to keep their house clean,
I worry about your life,
And if I'll see you turn sixteen.

Others can't stand the thought
Of paying bills and working every day,
I can't stand the thought,
I may not see your eighteenth birthday.

People may complain about
Things getting out of their hands
I am sad I may not get old,
And see you turn into a wonderful young man.

They may get annoyed and angry,
And say their ills are caused by someone,
I am angered by my shortened life,
And I may not see you turn twenty-one.

And they may worry about
Their priorities and getting through.
I don't want to sound selfish,
Nathan, I'll forever love you.

The treatment

To combat the sleepless nights and anxiety, my oncologist prescribed some Oxazepam. It was so strong for my body. There were some nights while taking this medication I felt like I stopped breathing and my heart rate would be so slow when I woke up from my latest nightmare. I expressed my concerns to the doctor and he assured me I wouldn't die from forgetting to breathe because of this medication. But the sensations were so real for me that I decided to stop taking it.

I continued on with life as best as I could, even though I felt like crap. I was so relieved to finish chemotherapy and was looking forward to getting back to a semi-normal kind of life. I had no idea the effects from the chemotherapy would remain in my system for such a long time afterwards. I still have lumps under my skin, have gained weight, and have tingling in my toes,[22] which I now know is called peripheral neuropathy. This also explains the dizziness I sometimes get or the strange feeling of not knowing where my body is in space, which occurs from time to time. Not forgetting the early onset menopause caused by the chemotherapy.

On February 2014, I went for my first MRI.[23] Not being a *patient* patient, I decided to investigate the scan myself before hearing the official report from my doctor. I noticed a red patch glowing on the scan in my spine. My breath caught in my throat when I spotted the anomaly. I knew from speaking with the oncologist there was a chance the cancer could go to my spine, my brain or my lungs. I thought the worst and cried for a week until my doctor's appointment. I walked in thinking I would be told I'd have to go through hell again but was assured the colouring was just normal bone degeneration, the osteoarthritis most people get as they age. The relief was unlike anything I'd experienced before. A massive sigh is an understatement. I promised myself I would not investigate for myself, but promises can be broken. I could never stop myself.

With no more chemicals being pumped through my body, I slowly began to regain my energy and strength. I continued to do the circuit training and I was feeling much better. I also began seeing a counsellor for trauma and loss counselling and spoiling myself with massages. I began working in the community as a personal carer – only a few hours a week, but it kept me busy.

Preparing to say goodbye

January 2014

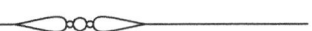

The words of the oncologist kept ringing in my ears – *Two years at best... Two years at best.* Even though my treatment was done, it felt like the clock was ticking down for me every single day. I'd already lived through seven months of those two years and it terrified me.

When I was given the terminal diagnosis by the oncologist, I was urged to get my affairs in order. I guess it made sense. Who would want to leave a mess behind when they go? I was no longer afraid of dying. My greatest fear was John would be unable to cope and Nathan would be without his mother and most of his aunties. Although John's sister, Aunty Chrissie, was still in his life, the distance would mean not catching up on weekends like we did when we lived in Melbourne. My sisters, niece and nephews had stopped all

I was no longer afraid of dying.

contact with me, and this loss had a negative effect on my mental health. It was an extremely challenging time, one that would take years to come to terms with. I knew my darling husband would come up against hurdle after hurdle if I didn't outline exactly how everything was to be done.

> *I decided to write a Dear John letter.*

I decided to write a Dear John letter of a very different kind. This letter would be read by my husband when I'd left this world. I never imagined I would be planning for my death at the age of forty-six.

Outlined in the letter was Nathan's routine through to the financials. I documented everything for John so he wouldn't be left in overwhelm. In a way, it was a relief to know all of this could be organised. If I were to be hit by a bus walking home, John would struggle to know what needed doing and when to do it. Although I really knew he would manage, this was mainly for my own sanity. Now, no matter what happened, he would be clued in to everything. I transferred the vehicle registration and insurances to John's name alone so he wouldn't have to deal with red tape and administration headaches in trying to access any of our accounts or pay the bills after I had died.

Ordinarily, I was someone who would step up and take charge, but I know my whole psyche changed in that time of my life. Everything became urgent. One day, painting a room in the house was of the utmost importance. The next, it would be buying Nathan a car so he had one of his own when he was old enough to drive.

I discovered Dr Colin Dicks, a radiation oncologist specialist, and his website Dying to Understand.[24] It was an incredible resource that enabled me to come to terms with what I needed to consider now I had a terminal diagnosis.

I figured it would be easy to plan my funeral as well. I called a funeral company and a gentleman with a softly-spoken voice advised me I would have to be over fifty to create a funeral plan. I informed him of my situation and he relented, allowing me the chance to lock in everything, from where I wanted my ashes to go after I was cremated through to which song they would feature at my funeral. (This changed so many times!) I marvelled at the irony of it all. *I'm doing all this planning and I won't get to join in the party. Why do I care what song they play? No one likes what music I listen to anyway.*

I was very frugal with what I organised. I wanted to leave as much money for my son as possible. I found that I had become quite self-absorbed in the process, thinking only about what I wanted. This became apparent when I told John I wanted my ashes to be placed in the wall next to my mum in Victoria.

"What about what I want?" came his simple reply.

I hadn't even considered the effects on his mental health. I realised it would be selfish If I were laid to rest in another state. John and Nathan wouldn't be able to visit me easily. I became more open in my communication with him. I guess part of me wanted to shield

> ***Thinking about your mortality can be confronting.***

him from the pain of it all. As anyone who has ever planned their wills and estates and had all of those really tough discussions, thinking about your mortality can be confronting. The fact that I had been given a rough estimate of two years to live only served to amplify every single emotion tied to this type of planning.

In a way, it's like you are planning for a holiday. You've got to think of everything in advance and organise and plan accordingly. Only you don't know when this holiday is actually going to happen.

This thought that the end could come at any time plagued me. I began taking precautions everywhere, including putting a plastic sheet underneath my usual bed linen in case I died during my sleep. I wanted to make it easy for everyone to clean up the mess. There were days when John thought I was going nuts. I was always in a hurry, like I was racing against the clock, and if something wasn't done *now* there was a danger it would never get done at all.

> **Easter bunnies and public holidays were more important.**

My fears were realised in March 2014, when I found a lump in my groin. It was no larger than a marble. It hadn't been picked up on the regular CT scans I had been having every three months as it was just a little below where the imaging stopped. Instead, I'd found it on one of the regular self-body checks I had done routinely following my kidney surgery. I figured I needed to be on high alert from then on in, and this discovery highlighted the importance of this even more.

I went to the doctor, who then referred me to the radiologist and a biopsy was performed. It would be another two weeks until I found out it was more of this killer cancer. I was absolutely devastated, believing the four months of chemo I had endured had all been for nothing.

What really annoyed me was that once we'd found and identified the cancer, I then had to wait a month before my course of radiation started. The only reason for the delay was the timing. I should have started radiation treatment the following week, but the regime of consistent treatment could not be enforced – Easter bunnies and public holidays were more important, apparently. I know it's just how things go sometimes, but I believed things just kept stacking up against me.

Radiation is often the next go-to after chemotherapy has done all it can do. I was prescribed a month of external-beam radiation, which is where you have to lie completely still for about fifteen minutes while a machine treats the area around the tumour.

> *I held still and visualised the radiation knocking out every one of those little bastard cancerous cells.*

It is a more concentrated and targeted approach, and the American Cancer Society explains that various machines use "high-energy particles or waves, such as x-rays, gamma rays, electron beams, or protons, to destroy or damage cancer cells".[25]

Just like chemo, the idea is to disrupt and kill cancer cells. Each time I entered the CT machine for the radiation treatments, I held still and visualised the radiation knocking out every one of those little bastard cancerous cells. Blasting them away. Each treatment, I would imagine there was a smaller and smaller amount of cancer in my body. It was the only thing that would take my mind away from the suffocating feeling of remaining deadly still for the required time as the machine drew me in under its canopy. I attended radiation treatment every day from the end of April 2014 up to my birthday in early June 2014. And just like the chemotherapy treatment, the knock-on effects happened later on. The targeted lymph nodes in which the cancer had taken hold were burnt and the burn spread further away to my leg and labia. My hair follicles had also been burned. The burn was like somebody had thrown hot water over me. I could hardly walk due to this pain. I later found the radiation also played havoc with my intestines, causing food to sometimes get stuck, which felt like a baby wearing footy-boots kicking in my belly. The bowel had become less pliable, causing strange sensations.

What are the odds?

April 2014

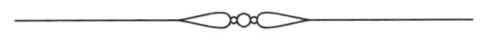

Physically, I was able to recover much quicker from the radiation than I had following chemo, and I bounced back relatively quickly. But, mentally, my mind was abuzz. *The cancer had come back. What if it comes back for a third time? What if it never stops coming back?* I doubted whether I would be able to sustain a level of positivity if this battle continued to rage within my body.

I'd had one 'all clear' scan following radiation. My oncologist never liked to use the word 'remission' because it is so often misinterpreted. I also believed I would never get to that stage.

Dr Laura Martin, former medical editor for WebMD, defines the two types of remission as:

1. **Partial remission** – the cancer is still there but your tumour has gotten smaller, or in cancers like leukaemia, you have less cancer throughout your body.
2. **Complete remission** – tests, physical exams, and scans show that all signs of your cancer are gone. However, this doesn't mean you are cured.[26]

Some doctors also refer to complete remission as NED (an acronym that stands for 'no evidence of disease'). The reason why doctors can never say you are cured is because there is no sure-fire way of knowing all of the cancer cells in your body have gone. There is potential, particularly in the first five years, for cancer tumours to reappear. My oncologist would simply say I had the 'all clear' following my regular CT scans, and I understood that this just meant 'this time around'. I am always quick to point this out to people and have never been fond of the word 'remission'. Especially since I was officially diagnosed as terminal, 'remission' felt like a bad word I could not allow myself to use.

I often found myself wondering if my predicament would have been different if I had a 'common' type of cancer, like breast cancer. Women diagnosed with breast cancer have incredible survival rates – in 2020, Australian Institute of Health and Welfare statistics show the chance of surviving at least five years following a breast cancer diagnosis was 91%.[27] The same timeframe for CDC saw only an 8.8% survival rate.[28]

Seeing those statistics did little to help my state of mind. I was a little jealous. Because the cancer I had was not common, little research was done, therefore little funding went to finding possible cures. It's surprising how many cancers are in the same predicament. A look at Rare Cancers Australia (RCA) shows just how many other rare and less common cancers there are. [29]

It's the green I need

August 2014

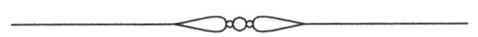

Traditional medicine had done all it could for me. I was literally in a 'wait and see' holding pattern. It was then that John and a girlfriend of mine suggested I look into cannabis oil as a possible way of improving my chances of a clean bill of health moving forward.

They told me it was being talked about as a medicine that could combat cancer. I was dubious at first – the sceptical side of me screamed, *What? Do they think I'm some kind of hippie?* I smiled and nodded at the suggestion. I was a huge critic of anything that proclaimed to be a miracle cure, and I still don't believe it is to this day. I gave John a few looks that said, *Are you crazy?* But as he seemed so sure, John ventured online to find out as much as he could about it and I soon found myself curious to learn more.

Do they think I'm some kind of hippie?

My only experience with anything related to cannabis was when I was a teen and I'd shared a joint with a few friends. I must confess, I'd also drunk about six stubbies of beer beforehand. I recall falling asleep on the couch and then waking up and realising I had to get home. I hated the feeling of not being in control and feeling drowsy and groggy. I rarely touched it again.

Explaining some terms...

There is so much confusion around the terms cannabis, hemp and marijuana, so here is a basic explanation of each and how they all fit together.

- **Cannabis** is a genus of flowering plants in the Cannabaceae family, which consists of three primary species: Cannabis sativa, Cannabis indica and Cannabis ruderalis.[30]

- **Hemp** is a term used to classify varieties of cannabis that contain 0.3% or less tetrahydrocannabinol (THC) content (by dry weight). It is also the strongest natural fibre in the world and is known to have more than 50,000 different uses, including home textiles, industrial textiles, building materials and body care.

- **Marijuana** is a term used to classify varieties of cannabis that contain more than 0.3% THC (by dry weight) and can induce psychotropic or euphoric effects on the user.

The cannabis plant has been used as a medicine for thousands of years, with burned cannabis seeds found in the graves of shamans in China and Siberia from as early as 500 BC.[31] Historians have traced cannabis from Central Asia before it made its way to Africa, Europe and the Americas, where hemp fibre was used to make clothing, paper, sails and rope as well as being used in food and in medicines.

What is interesting is that the early cannabis plants had very low levels of THC, which is the chemical responsible for cannabis's mind-altering effects.

It wasn't until the late 1920s that the criminalisation of cannabis was brought into effect in the United States and the stigma surrounding the plant was born. The release of the church-funded movie *Reefer Madness* in 1937 is a prime example of how they used fear to brainwash the idea that smoking cannabis would literally turn you into a crazy person who was partial to self-harm, sex orgies and criminal behaviour.[32] As more countries begin to decriminalise or even legalise recreational or medical cannabis, this stigma seems to remain intact, and this is something I will talk about later in the book.

> *This stigma seems to remain intact.*

One of the things I get asked all the time is what the difference is between cannabis oil and hemp seed oil. Hemp seed oil is readily available in many health food shops and some people get confused about what it is they are actually buying.

Hemp seed oil, often mislabelled as simply hemp oil, is a cold-pressed oil made from the seeds of the hemp plant.[33] It does have some health benefits in that it has plenty of essential fatty oils and you can easily buy it. On the other hand, true whole-plant oil derived from the cannabis plant is made from the buds/flowers of the female cannabis plant and comprises many different cannabinoids.

Of course, there were plenty of people out there who were spruiking cannabis oil as the miracle cure for cancer but I was never going to believe that. I was forever a sceptic and had to find things out for myself, not take anybody's word for it. I came across some incredibly in-depth resources that described the intricate endocannabinoid system we have in our bodies and how these systems react to certain components found within a cannabis plant.

I was elated when I uncovered that three years of investigations have shown that a modified form of medical cannabis can kill or inhibit cancer cells without impacting normal cells.[34] This new knowledge made a somewhat difficult decision much easier. I had nothing to lose.

> *I had nothing to lose.*

I was shocked that none of this had ever been discussed during my nursing course, even though I recall seeing the endocannabinoid system in one of my textbooks. It is all very complex, but I'd like to explain it at a surface level for you to gain a basic understanding of how it works. If you are inclined to find out more, check out the Additional Resources page at the end of this book.

What is the endocannabinoid system?

The endocannabinoid system (ECS) is a complex cell-signalling system inside the human body.[35] The system keeps your body stable and if something like pain from an injury throws your internal environment into chaos, the ECS kicks in to restore order.

The ECS has three core components: **endocannabinoids**, **receptors** and **enzymes**.

- **Endocannabinoids** are molecules made by your body and scientists have discovered two types: anandamide (AEA) and 2-arachidonoylglyerol (2-AG). Your body produces these molecules as needed and they travel around your body and connect to receptors to address certain ailments.

- The two main endocannabinoid **receptors** are CB1 receptors, which are mostly found in the central nervous system, and CB2 receptors, which are mostly found in your peripheral nervous system, especially immune cells.

- The **enzymes** are present to break down endocannabinoids once they've completed their task. For those of you who want the specifics: AEA is broken down by fatty acid amide hydrolase and monoacylglycerol acid lipase typically breaks down 2-AG.

What are cannabinoids?

Despite having a similar name to endocannabinoids, **cannabinoids** are the natural compounds found in the cannabis plant.[36] The major compounds cannabidiol **(CBD)** and tetrahydrocannabinol **(THC)** are probably the most misunderstood elements of the cannabis debate.

- **CBD** can be extracted from hemp or the Cannabis sativa plant.
- **CBD** is found in various hemp oils, supplements and extracts, whereas **THC** is the main psychoactive compound – it's the part that makes you high.

Both compounds are similar to the endocannabinoids in your body and are therefore compatible with the receptors. But they do have different effects.

- **CBD** is shown to help with anxiety, depression, inflammation, pain, nausea, migraines and seizures, whereas **THC** binds with the CB1 receptors in the brain to produce a high.
- **THC** helps with pain, muscle spasticity, glaucoma, insomnia, appetite boosting and anxiety.

Once I looked into cannabis oil as a medicine, a whole new world of possibility opened up to me. Being an open-minded person and very desperate, I was excited by this new possibility. John and I researched for hours on the internet.

I couldn't understand why the use of cannabis was such a taboo subject in some parts of the world and was devastated that Australia was among the countries that showed no signs of making it legal at that time in 2014.

In 2019, medical cannabis was finally legalised in Australia, with the caution that patients had to meet strict requirements to be eligible for a prescription. Even so, the cost is often prohibitive for people who are already struggling financially due to ill health. It seemed so unfair. Imagine if this could be freely available to the sick and dying.

Imagine if this could be freely available to the sick and dying.

I had been heartened by the research and anecdotes I had been seeing online, but there were two major concerns: none of the research had been done in Australia AND medical cannabis was illegal at the time. I felt like we were decades behind other countries on that front and the frustration often turned to anger when I thought about it.

Despite all of this, I decided I was going to give cannabis oil a try. At the time, it was a Schedule Two drug – in the same category as heroin – and, therefore, not something I could request from my specialist.

This is how I found myself in that alleyway in Nimbin.

John's research had found this was the place to go for anything to do with cannabis. We had recently bought a motorhome ready for an epic road trip around the country to make memories and bond as a family. Its maiden voyage was out to Nimbin – the infamous pot capital of New South Wales.

Here I was, a middle-aged woman on a mission to find an illegal substance that I hoped might save my life. Not the typical pothead. But put yourself in my shoes. I had tried the traditional and legal way and, as far as I knew, it wasn't working, so I was open to any and all possible solutions.

> **I felt like a criminal.**

With John remaining at a protective distance beside me as we walked through Nimbin, I found a dodgy office out the back of a decrepit alleyway and passed my details on to the person who said they had a contact for me, who would call me to put me onto some cannabis. It all felt so unnatural. They were also cautious of me. I felt like a criminal even asking the questions I needed to in order to get on the right track.

I wasn't able to find any cannabis oil to take home with me that night, but I did purchase a book called *A Grower's Guide*. It was an expensive book with a gold cover. But this was too scientific for my layperson's mind. It was a good read for the right person. I needed information quickly and to the point. This was not *the* book. I was not interested in becoming the drug lord of the Sunshine State, but I felt obliged to purchase something in their store as I didn't want to feel untrustworthy. I was given the contact number for a man whom I will call

Steve. It all sounded very mafia-like, which only added to my nervousness about the whole situation.

The evening after we came home, I received a call from Steve with details on how to access his website. Yes, he had a website I could order from! I was aware of Amsterdam having many websites and a ton of information. America too had a wealth of information and websites to order cannabis cookies and any food substances you might crave. But I couldn't believe my luck that from Australia, this country so far behind the rest of the world, Steve had a website I could connect with. I had no idea how he managed to get away with it, but I didn't really care.

It would have been hilarious if I was not in such a predicament. This was probably my last resort. It has taken me years to see the light-hearted side of this situation.

From the moment I placed the order, I had visions of the Australian Federal Police bashing in my door and whisking me away to jail. I was a fan of the show *Border Security* and I knew how thorough the screening process was for the postal system. I felt like a criminal when all I was trying to do was give myself the best chance at survival. Here I was, on a knife's edge, waiting for that highly anticipated parcel to arrive in my letterbox.

All I was trying to do was give myself the best chance at survival.

When the parcel arrived a month later without an accompanying guard of police officers, I breathed a nervous sigh of relief. I was also relieved Steve hadn't ripped me off. Then the rush of excitement came over me – time to get into it!

I started treatment that night. I carefully opened the package, tearing the paper away excitedly and cautiously. I did not want any of it to spill. I was deflated when I saw that this amber-coloured oil, which smelt like grass clippings, had seeped out a little onto the paper it was wrapped up in. The brown dropper bottle was so small. The pictures I saw on the internet had appeared to be much bigger. This small bottle of what I hoped was cannabis oil, which had cost me over one thousand dollars, was hopefully going to save my life. There was no way I was going to delay it for another second. To me, it felt like a life and death situation. I had zero time to waste.

I had an idea of how to take cannabis oil and how many drops at a time, thanks to a handy worksheet from the website. Using the dropper from the bottle, I was to allow the drops to sit under my tongue for as long as possible, absorbing slowly into my mouth cavity. However, when you buy illegal cannabis oil off the internet, you don't know what you're getting. The more I used it, the more the underside of my tongue began swelling up. I ended up with a lump half the size of a pea on my frenulum – the thing that connects your tongue to the bottom of your mouth. I don't know whether the alcohol had not been dissolved totally from the oil or whether there were some impurities in there. It is an incredibly hard position to be in when you have to trust people you have never met with your health. I didn't go to the supplier to complain as I had a fear of being blacklisted if I said anything to jeopardise our professional relationship. And I wasn't about to go to my GP and tell him about cannabis oil causing the painful inflammation.

Meanwhile, I was trying to tie up loose ends. I thought it would be great to go on some kind of holiday with my family to make some memories John and Nathan would hold dear forever. It would be the first time Nathan had left the country and it was the start of my plan to tick items off my bucket list. The voice of the specialist who had given me my diagnosis had rung in my mind at the most unexpected of times – *Make memories with your family while you can.*

My passport had expired, and until then, I hadn't seen the need to renew it. Since John and I had married in America, there was some rigmarole around getting my name legally changed on my passport. I'd been able to do it easily in other realms in my life – banks, driver's licence, electricity bills – but this was a little trickier. We got there in the end after lots of tears and finally some assistance from our local Member of Parliament.

A tropical getaway to The Naviti Resort in Fiji seemed like the perfect solution to break the monotony of living cancer every waking hour. We were fortunate that both John and I had invested in life insurance when we first became a couple. As we both knew, life throws all sorts of spanners. Now my life insurance payout, along with early access to my superannuation, was enabling us to pay the bills while I was unable to work. Pleasantly, it also gave us the ability to make lots of travel memories.

A few months later, I started to get hot flushes out of nowhere. I could feel them coming on. My heart began to race. I had a sense of urgency and felt irritation within my body, a bit like when you are desperate for the toilet. I felt a strange sensation – a wave of heat enveloped me and I wanted to take all my clothes off to cool down. But I knew once this passed I would be cold because the hot perspiration would become icy cold water on my skin. At night, I would sometimes sweat so much it made my wet night clothes stick to me.

> *I had early onset menopause.*

Unsure of what was happening, I went to the doctor to flag it as a concern. After a few minor examinations, I was told news I never expected… I had early onset menopause. It had been brought on by the chemotherapy.

To add insult to injury, chemo-induced menopause is more intense than the natural kind.[37] I am still dealing with the impacts of this as I write this book years later. It plays a big role in why I can't run as far as I used to. There are days when I can only get to the end of my street on a run and then be in a big pool of sweat from the hot flushes before my body's natural sweat response to running has a chance to kick in. It wears me out. As any woman who has had the 'joy' of experiencing menopause knows, it just comes at random times. You might not even be exerting yourself and it just happens… it's so annoying.

By August, I had done enough research to understand that in order for cannabis oil to become effective as a 'cancer killer', three drops a day must increase to the equivalent of one millilitre (ml) per day and that ml must be taken for forty continuous days. There was so much conflicting information on the internet. One site said forty drops was the magic number. I later found out that twenty-eight drops was equivalent to one ml, but I figured it couldn't do any harm to take too much rather than not enough. If anything, I would likely be drowsier. It was unlikely I would die from having too much. According to the National Drug & Alcohol Research Centre, no deaths were directly linked to cannabis toxicity but due to accidental injury.[38]

> *It was unlikely I would die from having too much.*

Counting how many drops of cannabis I was taking every day became a bit of a challenge. After the fourth day, I was losing count. I decided to keep a diary to keep me on track. I also used it to document how I was feeling and what I was doing.

The first day was easy – three drops over twenty-four hours. That would be one drop every eight hours. It took about half an hour for the THC to kick in. I was told I wouldn't get stoned, but I can tell you now, I did. What I found interesting was that it was a totally different 'stone' to the one I'd experienced when I was a teen, inhaling from a joint. I was able to function, I wasn't too drowsy and I still felt in control. That said, I chose not to drive a car and left all of the money-handling and other financial obligations to John, just to be on the safe side.

The effects didn't kick in right away, so the first time I took it, I took a little more, thinking I'd miscalculated the dosage. It was really bizarre to go from feeling completely fine one moment and then getting up to do something and having that outer-body feeling of having left your brain behind. I'd describe it as feeling spacey. I was worried about increasing the dosage slowly each day but found my body adapted as I went along.

I had taken prescription medications as I'd needed them throughout my life and I realised they would also have side

Everybody reacts differently to cannabis. effects. Even antihistamines cause me to have reduced coordination and slower reaction time. The fact that cannabis oil also caused some side effects was not surprising, even though most research indicates this is largely due to the cannabinoids in the oil reacting negatively with components of pharmaceutical medication patients are also taking.[39] Hence the time in my teens, when I had drunk a lot of alcohol before I experimented with a joint at a party. It was all clearer to me now. Alcohol was the drug.

Everybody reacts differently to cannabis as they do with all medications. I am no different. Some of the possible side effects include dry mouth, dry eyes, dizziness, anxiety, paranoia, lethargy, increased heart rate and decreased blood pressure.[40] I found I was more prone to feeling tired and having a dry mouth, which gave me the exact opposite of minty fresh breath. To me, this was a positive side effect, as it encouraged me to drink more water, just what my remaining kidney needed.

We have no trouble trusting our doctors and big pharmaceutical companies with medication that could potentially give side effects, but this same mindset doesn't seem to apply when it comes to cannabis oil. We still believe prescription medications are okay and must be safe to use if the government allows their use. Because prescriptions are legal, the side effects and their contraindications are a small price to pay for good health, right?

As I investigated further into research around cannabis oil,

I found there are three main types of cannabis strain – sativa, indica and ruderalis – and they each have unique qualities. Hybrids and different varieties for each of these strains are produced and can help with a number of health issues.[41] There are hundreds of sub-types of each of the two main strains too, each having different percentages of CBD and THC within their make-up. I found a website overseas which broke down these percentages and also showed whether the seeds were sativa or indica – important for the ailments being treated.[42]

Different strains and hybrid species give you varying levels of THC and CBD. With a greater understanding of how the strains worked, I spent countless hours researching cannabis plants in order to see if I could procure the main ingredient to begin to make my own cannabis oil. It was only a thought at that stage, something I believed would save me money.

The main cannabis strains

- **Cannabis sativa** often produces a 'mind high' or an energising, anxiety-reducing effect. If you use sativa-dominant strains, you may feel productive and creative, not relaxed and lethargic. Some strains can treat fatigue, stress, nausea, acute pain, mental fog, anxiety, PTSD, depression, migraine and glaucoma.

- **Cannabis indica** is sought after for its intensely relaxing effects. It may also reduce nausea and pain and increase appetite. Some strains can treat chronic pain, muscle spasms, insomnia, low appetite, PTSD, restless leg syndrome, inflammation, stress and mood disorders.

- **Cannabis ruderalis** isn't routinely used for medicinal or recreational/therapeutic purposes because of its low THC potency.

I felt a keen sense of dismay and frustration that I was spending the precious little time I thought I had left trying to access something that could potentially prolong my life. I would much rather have been doing something I enjoyed. Not researching. When I did find information, a lot of it was the author's own opinion and point of view. Once I saw the word 'cured' I dismissed the information. I find it unacceptable that people can make such claims as this. I did not want people to be so one-sided and closed to other opinions. We call our country 'free', but it still appears to be lacking free speech and information on such subjects. *Why isn't this just available to people? It's a natural bloody product!*

On one occasion a friend gave me some seeds, but I didn't know what strain they were and decided to source some I could be more certain of. I loved gardening and had a little bit of a green thumb, but I was not, for the life of me, able to grow cannabis. I bought endless numbers of books to read so I could find out how to grow them successfully. This was just another thing that was taking up my extremely valuable time. In the end, I found a website that sold seeds in a country where cannabis was legal. They were able to send three indica seeds sewn discreetly into some clothing. I was in a state of pure desperation and I went ahead with it. The business I bought from were incredibly helpful with their advice and support – it was a legitimate business in that country – and, once again, I felt frustrated that it had to be so hush-hush in Australia.

> *I felt frustrated that it had to be so hush-hush.*

Now the real challenge had arrived – I had to grow these plants as quickly and efficiently as possible. It was extremely hard to find credible information about how to grow a cannabis plant. Even in countries where it was legal, I found just about every website contradicted the one I'd read before. It was difficult to cut through the noise (and a waste of hours) and determine the best way to cultivate these three precious little seeds.

I soaked my three seeds in a jar of water until they cracked, then put them on tissue paper and waited for the taproot to pop through. All three seeds were starting to take and I did a little happy dance when I saw the third shoot appear. I planted the seeds in three peat pots and waited for them to emerge through the soil. Only one did. I was a little deflated by this but clung to the hope this one little plant provided me. I treasured this plant for three months, and took a cutting from it and learned how to clone. During the fourth month, just before it was ready to be harvested, I noticed a lot of ants trailing up and down the main stem. This concerned me and I took to social media to find out how to stop the ants from potentially devouring my plant before I could reap the rewards of my months of nurturing.

Putting my faith in social media information turned out to be the biggest mistake I could have made. After an hour of researching natural ant killers, I used a ratio of 50:50 vinegar and water. One day later, my plant was dead.

At least you still have the cutting! I tried to tell myself to lighten the mood, but the fact was it would be another three months before this one was mature. I was so angry that my indica medicine was dead. Furious even. This would mean a costly delay in my cannabis oil treatment.

Unable to simply duck down to the doctors to ask for another option, I began trawling the internet for any aspect of hope. I was growing more upset and frustrated every time I saw how some other countries around the world had legalised cannabis oil and it would have been a breeze for me to access the medicine I needed without all of the sneaking around and exorbitant expenses of the black market.

John and I actually spoke about moving over to America to live, in order to gain access to cheaper cannabis oil. There is no doubt it would have been more cost-effective for me to receive my ongoing treatment in the US, and the idea that I wouldn't have to hide and feel ashamed of using cannabis oil seemed liberating. But the costs of moving over there meant it was not an option for us. It really was a shitty situation.

I almost leaped out of my chair with joy when I found a company selling cannabis oil, but when I requested a price list from them, I was deflated when I saw they were offering a tincture. In a nutshell, tinctures are concentrated herbal extracts made by soaking components of a plant in alcohol or vinegar.[43]

> *John and I actually spoke about moving over to America.*

Through the copious research I had done, I knew the difference between true cannabis oil and a tincture, but I worried for all of the people out there who might not know they were not getting the proper medicine by ordering from this company or others like it. I wondered, *Who really had the time to learn the difference between putting cannabis under lights, going with a hydro set-up or sticking with the more traditional bush cannabis growing methods?*

In the midst of all of the angst over my plants, I was pleased that I was still kicking along in November 2014. So, I planned a trip to New Zealand. I chose to up the ante and we booked a fourteen-day cruise around the land of the long white cloud. I couldn't take my dwindling supply of cannabis oil with me on holiday. I really didn't want my small screen debut to be on *Border Patrol!* I took some time to make peace with the fact that I would have to have a break from my treatment while we were away. I really didn't want to get caught and ruin what could very well be our last family holiday.

This was more of the type of holiday I had visions of when thinking about what my ideal last holiday would look like. We stayed in a mini-suite, which doubled the price but it meant Nathan could stretch out in a full-sized bed and there was a nice big bed for John and me. It had a spa and a balcony so we had plenty of fresh air, and it was a beautiful space to chill out in if we didn't want to head out that day.

Nathan was right into the world of Tolkien and *The Hobbit* movie had not long been released, so we did everything Hobbit-related while we were in New Zealand. He had the best time, and it was an absolute joy to see his face light up when we went to the various movie locations and saw some of the props from the movies.

Making memories

December 2014

Nathan had just finished Year Nine and wasn't doing very well with his grades, so John and I decided to homeschool him for the next year or two. Just a few months later, we made another decision – to pack up the motorhome and travel. The idea was to take on all of Australia, but our first leg would see us head back to Melbourne to see friends and family and then spend time in Tasmania. The rest we would figure out as we went along.

We set off for Goondiwindi, on the border of Queensland and New South Wales, in December 2014. I was so excited about the trip. I'd contacted friends to catch up with as we went along.

I remember Goondiwindi being extremely hot and I was constantly bothered by mosquitoes and flies, but it was so good to be on our way for this adventure. Nathan took up residence in the captain's bed above the driver's seat, and John and I were to share the bed you make up at the back of the cabin. Making that bed was like putting a complicated jigsaw puzzle together. I found out that the mattress for the bed had different density of foam depending on where you were on the mattress. It was not the most comfortable bed in the world and if I had my time again, I'd bring my own mattress along with me!

The next stopover was in Dubbo, New South Wales, where we met up with Gary and Barb, the couple who had introduced John and me on that blind date years ago. We stayed at a holiday park with them. We were in our motorhome, and Gary and Barb were in their camper trailer. Our set of wheels wasn't the easiest thing to get around in, so we ended up walking to Dubbo Zoo from the caravan park and it was ridiculously hot. How I didn't pass out I'll never know.

We were so exhausted by the time we reached the zoo. I was relieved to see they had golf carts for hire to get around the huge complex, so we grabbed a couple and zipped around to all of the exhibits. We spent two nights there before moving on to West Wyalong. On the way, we got a puncture. Being the sturdy man of our house on wheels, John got out the jack and began cranking it up to lift the wheel off the ground. He'd already taken the wheel nuts off and placed them on the ground, with sweat dripping off him as he cranked and cranked. He had to stop every few seconds to swat away the flies that seemed to gravitate towards his head and nostrils. It wasn't long before he lost his patience. He knelt down to get better leverage on the jack and swore as what he thought was a stone from the gravel shoulder of the roadside was digging painfully into his knee. He picked up the offending object and flung it into the grass beside the road.

A few seconds after it had left his hand, he realised he'd just chucked away one of the wheel nuts! While replacing the tyre, he also noticed both the inside wheels on the dual wheel set-up at the back of the motorhome were bald. The sneaky buggers who'd sold us the motorhome had put new tyres on the outside and left the crappy ones on the inside. It was hard to see any tread on them and I doubted they were even legal. This drew more colourful language from John.

We slowed our driving pace right down because we were minus one wheel nut and worried about the wheel coming off and paranoid about the bald tyres. The place we had hoped would be able to help us in Wyalong was already closed, so we limped on at 70km an hour to Wagga. We made it there just before 5pm and they were able to fit two new tyres. They couldn't do anything about the wheel nut, which John was now feeling rather sheepish about. We stayed overnight in a caravan park. I had the bright idea that we would stay in one of the cabins there to have a break from the confines of the motorhome.

The moment we opened the door to the cabin, I regretted that decision. I couldn't stand the fact that it smelled of stale cigarettes with discarded cigarette butts all over the place – not the best environment for a reformed smoker like me. The single room had inbuilt bunk beds and a double bed below a leaky air conditioning unit. There was no way in hell Nathan was going to fit into one of the tiny bunk beds so Nathan and I stayed in the motorhome while John stayed in the cabin. It was the first night on our trip that I was able to sleep through the night because I didn't have John snoring his head off!

The following morning, we drove to Albury and had breakfast at a cafe before hitting the road once more, heading for Dandenong to see friends I had grown up with. I was so excited to finally be back in Victoria. We watched an outdoor movie, *Hercules*, that night, and I caught a cold, which put a dampener on things for me. Now that we were in Melbourne, we hired a Rent-a-Bomb car so it would be easier to get around. We also used this as an opportunity to exchange the mattress we had been sleeping on for a much better one, which was a million times more comfortable.

Nathan was relieved we made it to John's mum's place just before Christmas. He was totally over the motorhome and had ripped one of the curtains around his bed off the rail during one of his meltdowns. He was going stir-crazy. The timing was perfect for us to park where there were plenty of things around us to entertain him.

On Christmas Day, we went to Chrissie's friend's place for lunch with a huge gathering of family and friends. Dinner on Boxing Day was around the table at my mother-in-law's. It was beautiful to be surrounded by family once again. My own family had drifted off and we barely spoke now, so to feel the love around these tables with John's family was truly special.

We drove by our old home in Narre Warren and when I saw how run-down the area had become, I felt a rush of gratitude that we no longer lived there. I was deeply connected to my home on the Sunshine Coast and couldn't imagine still living in this part of the world. True to Melbourne weather, we experienced four seasons in one day, but it was great to be able to connect with old friends, some of whom I hadn't seen for many years. There were plenty of laughs.

Making memories

New Year's Eve was a cloudy day but, despite the skies, there were better moods all round in the motorhome. We drove to Station Pier, had chocolate shakes and iced coffee, and hung out all afternoon waiting to board the *Spirit of Tasmania*.

We met up with our friends Kellie and Peter, who were all set to spend a month with us on Australia's Apple Isle. We had packed my supply of cannabis oil into the back of the unplugged freezer in the motorhome, along with the empty capsules. I figured two oldies and their son would be less likely to be searched by any potential sniffer dogs than a group of young twenty-somethings travelling in a Kombi van but, then again, I was only assuming.

My heart was racing with panic when we pulled the motorhome onto the *Spirit of Tasmania* and were directed into a parking space. I was paranoid for the entire trip, always wondering if people were looking at me. *Is that a cop over there? Does he know what we've done? Can people smell it on me?* I had already planned how I was going to navigate the situation if it was discovered. I'd just tell them the truth. I figured it might be enough to save me from getting a criminal record if push came to shove.

We made it across the Tasman Sea without any issues and I breathed a lot easier once we'd pulled off the ferry at 6am on New Year's Day and started making our way to the campsite. We were twenty minutes en route to Cradle Mountain when we realised we hadn't stocked up on supermarket supplies. By the time we got to the site, Kellie and Peter had already set up their tent. I was in awe when a wild echidna scuttled by our motorhome as we were getting settled in. I stared at this marvel of nature and fully immersed myself in the moment. I knew this might be the only time I would be able to see this. John and Nathan weren't nearly as excited as I was. I simply stopped and watched the little echidna as it went on its merry way, totally oblivious to the hustle and bustle we were going through to set up camp.

I was in awe when a wild echidna scuttled by our motorhome.

Having ordered enough cannabis oil to last me for a fair while, I had decided to follow treatment protocol while we were travelling. The supplier had explained what I would have to endure – I called it the bombardment treatment. Essentially, it was about building up the number of drops of cannabis oil I was taking under the tongue to forty drops over the course of a day and continuing the treatment for a total of eighty days.

The theory behind it was that it was a ruthless assault on the cancer cells. Flooding the body with cannabis oil would deliver a type of shock treatment to the cancer cells with the aim of stopping them in their tracks. In medical terms, this is known as apoptosis.[44] I thought it was a very similar approach to traditional medicine's use of chemotherapy – the chemicals and processes flood your body and smash the cancer cells. Unfortunately, as I'd experienced, this was not friendly towards healthy body cells – it was brutal to them.

Now that I had a better understanding of the endocannabinoid system, it made sense to me to give it a try and I chose to start it while we were in Tasmania, where no one other than our travelling companions knew me.

My cannabis diary

- Day 1 to 3: One drop three times a day
  (total three drops over the day)
- Day 4 to 6: Two drops three times a day (6)
- Day 7 to 10: Three drops three times a day (9)
- Day 11 to 14: Four drops three times a day (12)
- Day 15 to 18: Five drops three times a day (15)
- Day 19 to 22: Six drops three times a day (18)
- Day 23 to 26: Seven drops three times a day (21)
- Day 27 to 30: Eight drops three times a day (24)
- Day 31 to 34: Nine drops three times a day (27)
- Day 35 to 38: Ten drops three times a day (30)
- Day 39 to 42: Eleven drops three times a day (33)
- Day 43 to 46: Twelve drops three times a day (36)
- Day 47 to 80: Thirteen drops three times a day (39)

This was what the game plan was supposed to look like, but I ended up really confused. How do you divide three into forty? I'd planned to make it forty-two, but with my brain not behaving the way it normally does, it was easier just to do thirty-nine drops a day. This meant thirteen drops three times daily and it was so much easier to keep track of.

As the bombardment progressed, I felt increasingly positive and tried to imagine myself beating the cancer. Every time I put those drops into by body, I visualised the oil's ingredients spreading throughout my bloodstream – *It's going to kill these little bastards and I will be good.* I was all in and I had nothing to lose.

The more cannabis oil I took, the sleepier I became. It was common for me to retire to the motorhome once or twice a day for a lie down. What I also noticed was that everything seemed calmer. I felt like there was nothing that could really bring me down. When we were driving along, I would giggle when the motorhome hit a bumpy patch and I was very content. The stress and worries that had plagued me since 2013 were non-existent. I had ensured I'd paid up all of the bills and taken care of everything before we left the Sunshine Coast so that I could focus on being present with my son and husband, and not make bad judgements on important matters.

We stayed at Cradle Mountain in early January 2015, walking around the lake on the Dove Circuit boardwalk and checking out the cascading river and magical old-growth rainforest in the Enchanted Walk along the edges of Pencil Pine Creek. It was in these beautiful surrounds that I was able to see a wombat in its native habitat. It was so cute! I loved listening to the sounds of the wildlife in the forest. It was like I had been transported back in time, surrounded by all those tall and sturdy trunks and not a whisper of civilisation outside of our small group.

John and I quickly discovered that motorhome living was not ideal for our tall son. He struggled to get comfortable in the bed and the longer we stayed away from home, the more frustrated he became at not having access to his video games. With Nathan's tensions running high and all of us suffering from cabin fever from time to time, it didn't take much for Nathan and John to be at loggerheads with one another once again. I tried my best not to let it get the better of me and I managed to block most of it out, only stepping in when a peacekeeper was required. I'd had visions of us travelling all around Australia in our motorhome, but I realised that my expectations were too high. We weren't cut out for that type of lifestyle.

Still, we soldiered on to complete our month in Tasmania and moved to St Helens on the north-east coast of Tasmania. We arrived at about 6pm after getting lost when the navigation system on our tablet lost signal and couldn't direct us. We were all in various states of frustration by that stage. Nathan wasn't helping me to set up camp and John had cracked a beer and simply sat down. I decided to remove myself from the situation and went to the beach. As I walked along the waterline with my bare feet in the sand, soft waves washed over the tips of my toes as the waves ebbed and flowed. I distanced myself from everything and began to think about my mortality. It wasn't a conscious decision; my mind simply took me there. Whenever I chose to think about my diagnosis and the cannabis oil I was taking, I only ever had positive thoughts around it. *I am beating this cancer. This oil will keep more tumours away. I can see the cancer cells wasting away.* It helped me immensely because being in an existential mindset was definitely not my normal.

After two hours, I went back to the campsite and lay down to sleep. But the unconscious thoughts took over my dreams. They were very different to the ones I allowed myself to think.

You'll be gone soon. What will happen to Nathan? Will John be able to cope? What is the meaning of life anyway? Why are we here? This is the last holiday I'll ever have – why are we doing it this way?

The mind is powerful. The next day it was hard to return to the carefree self I had been up to that point of the trip. To fight off the random thoughts of the day before and not dwell on them. Early on in my health journey, I had realised that you can either cry about shit or you can just try and enjoy what you have left. I was just trying to create memories and have a good time. It lights me up whenever Nathan remembers stuff from any of our holidays. He'll sometimes pipe up with, "Oh, I loved that cruise. I'm so lucky to have gone on those holidays." That is what I was aiming for: to give him some good memories rather than just being at home doing nothing and getting in each other's faces all of the time.

Of course, I hadn't seen the results of this time we were spending together just then; we were still in the thick of making these memories together. I decided to pull myself out of this spiral and change my mindset. I felt a little better once I had some food in my belly. John, Nathan and Peter went to play golf, and Kellie and I went grocery shopping, coming back for coffee and cake.

John had been sleeping in the tent since we set up at Cradle Mountain and there was a passing storm one night when John's quilt got saturated by the storm. We were fortunate to have powered sites and Kellie turned her tent into a little drying tent by putting the fan heater in there. She just made it really

Making memories

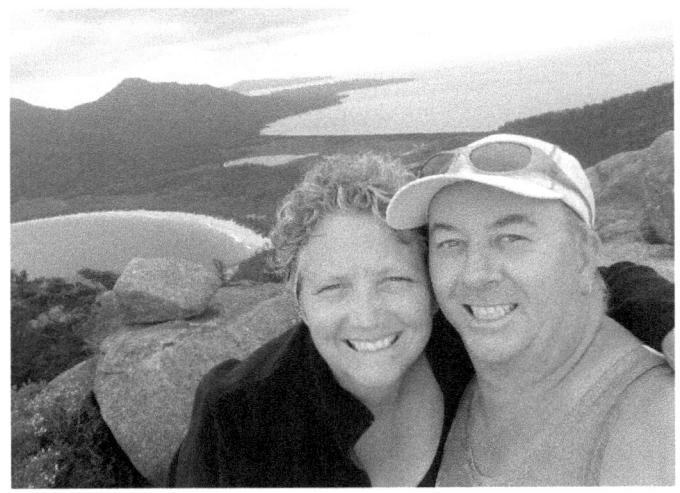

The summit of Mt Amos in Freycinet National Park, Tasmania

nice and toasty in there and then stuck the doona inside. We checked out the Bay of Fires and by the time we got back, John's bedding was completely dry.

We went to Wineglass Bay and then up to the lighthouse. Kellie and Peter suggested John and I go out and do something on our own the following day while they watched Nathan. I could count the number of times we'd been able to do that on one hand by that stage, and Nathan was then fifteen years old. Time together as a couple had been an absolute luxury since we had become parents.

We decided to use this precious time to climb Mt Amos together. The climb was no easy feat. There were sections where you

Time together as a couple had been an absolute luxury since we had become parents.

had to scoot along on your bottom because it was so steep, but once we got to the top, we were rewarded with an absolutely stunning view of Wineglass Bay. We then went out to an oyster restaurant and tried many different versions of oysters – I was surprised Kilpatrick was not the only variant! It was so lovely to not be pressured into leaving the restaurant in a hurry, which usually happened once Nathan finished eating. It was also a rarity for us to be able to enjoy each other's company as a couple and not as Mum and Dad.

We had some interesting times during our month in Tassie. We stayed for seven nights at the Airport Tourist Park in Hobart and, although it was a new venue at the time, there wasn't much to do around the campground so we had to fill our days with things to do elsewhere. We went to Richmond Gaol, Mount Wellington and Port Arthur, where we did what all tourists do and braved a ghost tour.

We quickly found out the campground was in a bit of a wind tunnel. We received a call from the park owners while we were all out on a day trip to let us know Kellie and Peter's tent had been blown away in a gust of wind whipped up by a storm. "Your tent has been compromised," were the exact words the caravan park owners used when delivering the news. It would have been comical if it wasn't so serious. The tent had been completely torn before being blown off its tethers. To their credit, the owners had salvaged all of the gear they could find and stored it safely until we returned. Kellie and Peter stayed in a cabin after that.

The horrid weather, the lost tent, almost running out of fuel on the way home the night before (I still don't remember

Making memories

how we managed to make it back to camp) and continuous bickering between John and Nathan was too much for me to handle. Tensions were running high at the camp site and I was at breaking point. I made the decision to walk away and try to get myself back to being grounded.

Because bad luck seems to come in waves, I was quick to see our current wave wasn't ready to head back out to sea just yet. Nathan had finally plucked up the courage to start using the caravan park ensuite attached to our site. It was a big deal for him because it had always given him anxiety. Even though he hated using the motorhome toilet because of the awful aroma, it was always a dilemma to use the park facilities and either John or I had to go with him. He summoned the courage to use the disabled toilet but he forgot to lock the door behind him. He was in the middle of his business when a man walked in. Nathan was totally freaked out and it was as if that one incident took him back a thousand steps in his progress, which was just awful for him.

The following day, it was Nathan's birthday and John and I presented him with a big decorative sword that looked like it could have come from the set of *The Hobbit* movie. He didn't show appreciation of it because it wasn't authentic. Nathan seemed to be able to identify whether something seemed out of place. The sword was nothing like the one in any of the Hobbit movies. Another trait of autism.

We checked out the Harley Davidson pub in Prospect Vale and went on a Segway rainforest tour at Hollybank on the off-road Segways. I was amazed that Nathan seemed to be able to ride the Segway with ease but has never caught on how to ride

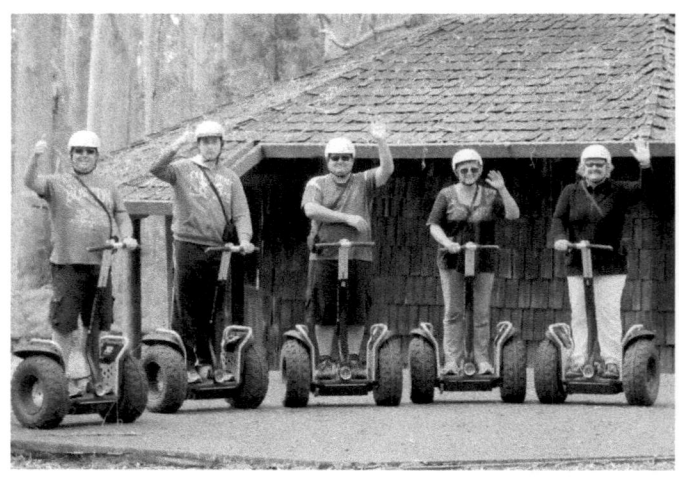

Hollybank off-road Segway tours were a nice way to finish our tour of Tassie

a normal bicycle. The tour was really fun; however, I was the one lagging behind the whole way.

It was so nice for all of us to be having a great time together and I began to forget about the crappy few days we'd just had. It was the perfect way to round out this section of our trip, as the next morning, we were packed and waiting once more for the *Spirit of Tasmania*. Along our travels, we were amazed at how opium farms were so visible from the road and legally grown for pharmaceutical companies. I could not make sense of this, given that growing cannabis for medicinal purposes was illegal.

Once we made it back over the Tasman and onto the mainland, we headed to East Gippsland and back to my

> *I think a lot of people don't like talking about death.*

hometown of Sale. I was able to catch up with friends in Rosedale and Heyfield. It was surreal to see so many of these people again, under the circumstances. It's hard to truly capture what that was like, but if I try – I felt like a broken record after a while. I just wanted them to know they had been a valued part of my life, and how I appreciated and loved them for being a part of it in the past.

It wasn't all doom and gloom. I felt really happy to be reconnecting with people and my health wasn't the sole topic of conversation. I think a lot of people don't like talking about death. But I was quite happy to answer questions or talk about it with those who wanted to know more. I found that the longer I'd known these friends, the more open they were to asking me the hard questions. I think when you're in my position, you've got a right to talk about it.

When you're in my position, you've got a right to talk about it.

I struggle to remember what it felt like to do that over and over again. Back then, I would have been a lot more emotional about it. But now, probably because my outcomes have been positive, it's hard to imagine how I was. It depends on how close my friends were, I suppose, as to how many tears I shed with them. How people reacted to the news was a mixed bag. Some people were warm and open and have kept in touch with me ever since. It seemed like no time had passed since I last saw some of my friends. Catching up with a friendly introduction was easy. Even though I may not had spoken to them for years, many of them had not changed.

It was on this leg of the journey I caught up with my brother. He gave me a hug. We hadn't been in touch for longer than I could remember – he never was a great communicator. It was usually one-sided. I haven't spoken to him since that day. I think he must think I am dead. Families aren't always what they are cracked up to be.

> **Families aren't always what they are cracked up to be.**

When we reached Woy Woy, I caught up with a dear friend who was a pothead from way back. I remember she had attempted to make some cannabis oil when I was about seventeen. It had the consistency of Vegemite. I thought we would have some roaring conversations about how I was so anti-dope and now I was dosing myself up on cannabis oil every day. But I quickly realised that our perceptions on the drug were very different.

When I asked her if she had any indica she shrugged her shoulders and looked utterly confused by my question.

"I don't know what you're taking there. I just use the bush stuff." She suggested putting a raw egg at the bottom of the pot before putting the seedling in it. Now I was totally confused, with some more information that didn't make sense.

It really showed me how little some recreational/therapeutic users understood the potential of the cannabis plant. If they didn't grasp it, how would people who have steered well clear of cannabis know?

The next stop was Darlington Beach in January 2015. It was here that I decided I would start to crochet a blanket for Nathan.

It would be a keepsake he could have with him forever. A little reminder of how much I loved him. Yeah, it was a bit sentimental and mushy, but I wanted to do little things that would keep me alive in his memory. When we'd visited an antique shop in Tasmania, I'd bought a book and had started to write down things from my family history and stories about when Nathan was young. While writing this book, I was cleaning out his room and found that book of family stories to show Nathan. He didn't show the slightest bit of interest in it. His ASD means he's not an overly emotional young man, but I've put all of these things away for safekeeping just in case he changes his mind later on.

While on our way back up the east coast to the Sunshine Coast, I received a phone call from a lady called Lynette Maguire. She asked me if I remembered entering a competition a month or so earlier. I was completely honest when I said I didn't even recall I'd done that. Some aspects of my life had become a complete blur since the diagnosis. This seemed to get her even more excited as she declared that **I'd won a wedding.** Lynette's charity, My Wedding Wish,[45] gifts weddings and vow renewal ceremonies to couples where one of the partners has a terminal diagnosis.

I'd never won anything in my life and I was taken aback by the enormity of it all. It felt amazing to have something to look forward to and to have that sprinkling of luck. After a meeting with Lynette when we arrived back home, our date was locked in. I was hugely excited to have something to plan and look forward to.

Pleading with a drug dealer

February 2015

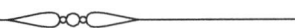

Ringing someone who is supplying you with an illegal substance to question their business skills is not likely to go well for you.

I found that out the hard way.

I had placed another order through Steve's website and made payment online, just as I had the previous times. Only this time, my nerve-riddled wait for the package stretched on… and on… and on. I began to panic, thinking it had been seized by sniffer dogs and police were already working to try to track down both me and the source of the package. John talked some sense into me after a few days where anxiety gripped every cell in my body.

"Give him a call, Alli!" he said in exasperation as I began spouting another 'what if…' scenario to my husband.

I want to make it clear it was most definitely not a case of me turning into a strung-out junkie climbing the walls waiting for their next fix. It was pure frustration at having to rely on someone else for this, combined with the worry that my cancer might return if there was a break in my cannabis oil treatment.

To say it was an awkward phone conversation is putting it mildly. I cut straight to the chase, giving him the date we placed the order and confirming payment had been made, just like I would have with any other business.

"Well, I haven't got the money," he stated.

I was trying my best to keep my cool, but inside I was fuming. I could see the predicament I was in here. He could say whatever he wanted and there was nothing I could do about it. *Who would I go to? The ACCC? The police? How could I report a case of being ripped off when the product was illegal?* He knew he had me and it made me furious.

> **I never thought I would see the day I'd be ghosted by a drug dealer.**

I said I would send him a screenshot of the money being transferred to his account from mine and he accepted the money had indeed been paid.

"So, where do you think my package is then?" I asked, trying my best to colour my tone with a little politeness.

He then said he had posted it the following day after I had paid him. He sent me a screenshot of the package delivered.

When I received the photo of the addressed parcel, I flipped out. The addressee's name started with an A, but that's exactly where the similarities to my details ended. This person had an Asian surname and the parcel was sent to Victoria!

I messaged him straight back declaring those were not my details and asked him to please send through my product, which I had paid about $1000 for. I never heard from him. The parcel never arrived. My money was never returned. I was never again able to contact Steve. I never thought I would see the day I'd be ghosted by a drug dealer. Yet, there I was, completely devastated that the one person I had come to rely on for my medicine was now unavailable and unwilling to help.

Remember, I had come into this realm of cannabis oil as a complete novice. Having this initial supply from Steve definitely helped me to breathe easier, knowing I had a source I could use while I educated myself even more. Back then, the only way to access any 'how to' instructions of any kind was on YouTube. There were many videos on the platform showing different methods of how to make your own cannabis oil at home, which was something I desperately wanted to do. The researching of videos was a time-consuming hassle. A hassle I really didn't want. But I didn't want to have to rely on someone else, nor did I have the energy to try to uncover someone else who could step into his role now that we had essentially been blacklisted in the black market.

> *We had essentially been blacklisted in the black market.*

I watched video after video – my browsing history would have been interesting that month! But I couldn't shake the fear that I could blow the roof off my house if I tried to make cannabis oil on my own. As if by some kind of divine intervention, a workshop on how to make cannabis oil appeared on my radar.

I kid you not! This workshop was to be held in a pub in Brisbane, so John and I ventured down to the city to see if I could become a more competent drug cook.

I stalled at the door when I looked inside and saw a small gathering of people, some much younger than John and I, but some much older too. Some of them were sporting dreadlocks or tie-dyed shorts or pants and my mind immediately jumped to the stereotype, *Look at these bloody hippies*. But most of them were normal looking. But I didn't know a single one of them. I didn't know what sort of health problem they may have been battling or what their reason was for being there. I told myself off for being so quick to judge, to fall into the trap of propping up the stigma I was working so hard to dispel. *You may have more in common with these people than you think.*

John and I had got a little lost trying to find the place, so we'd turned up a little late. Of course, this meant the only seats available were right at the front and centre of the room where nobody sits. I took a deep breath and walked through the door. Once I was inside, I saw there were more people than I had first thought. We had to walk past everyone and take pride of place right in the thick of the action, much to my dismay. At least I could see everything.

Once the presentation started, it didn't take long for me to relax. The information they were providing was practical and they took us step-by-step through different processes of making cannabis oil. We were able to see the Ice Water Extraction Method (also known as the Freezer Method) and the Evaporation Method. They also showed us how to use a still. I don't want to mention what type of still here in case they are removed from store shelves, like extraction fluid was once people (and the forces that be) realised it was also used in the process. Of course, they were using pretend plant matter, but I was able to see first-hand how it was all done and when it came to question time, nothing was off limits.

I felt reassured that there were many more people out there just like me, who were battling so hard to find credible information to follow. Many others in that room were wanting to treat a terminal or chronic illness that had consumed their lives. I felt liberated to be able to have this conversation in a public place with people from all walks of life. To feel supported in this educational environment. How they were able to pull this off when medical cannabis was still illegal is beyond me, but I was so grateful to have had the experience.

Safety first

May 2015

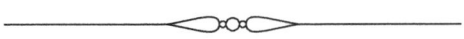

Now that Australians have access to medical cannabis oil through prescriptions, I don't recommend anyone try to create their own cannabis oil at home. But in 2015, this wasn't a reality for me. After leaving the workshop, I had a lot more confidence and decided I would give a couple of methods that were shown to me at the workshop a try.

Tincture is a mix of fluid and product left to ferment. The tincture[46] is then placed on a tray in a dust-free environment. Evaporation occurs and the residue remains. This was my very first attempt, and I am sure I didn't do it the correct way. To me, it seemed the safer way to go, but it was also the most expensive of the three options. The residue left at the end of the process becomes the medication. I was prepared to take this step so I could have peace of mind, knowing that I wouldn't be able to blow anything up. There is so much information available, usually from overseas websites. I also had to overcome the fact that a lot of ingredients were not easily available off the shelf or were called different things.

After that batch of oil had nearly been consumed, I ordered $1,200 worth of cannabis and set up equipment to make my oil a different way. This way was much better. This was the method that could end up with fire engines in my street! I had someone who, for this exercise, I will refer to as 'my friend'. My friend had experience with making cannabis oil. As he was a friend, I asked him to come to my house and go through the process with me. I was then able to learn hands-on. I should add that even finding the equipment was a mission. I was able to use a vessel and I found a shop that sold natural extraction fluid. Even though the fluid was a shelf item, the shop owner warned me not to tell anyone where I'd got it from. "Keep that hidden!" he warned me. "If the police pull you over, you didn't get that from me." It's hard to obtain extraction fluid now, but you can readily buy a bottle of isopropyl, which, when diluted with water, can be used on skin as an antiseptic. The product is also volatile, a flammable form of alcohol, and is easily available from major hardware stores. It is the stuff that will blow the roof off your house!

With every piece of equipment I bought, I was able to learn a little bit more about what I was doing and the safest way to do it. You can find help out there if you just look around, but it would have been better if I didn't have to do that. The saying 'life's too short' had taken on a whole new meaning for me and I felt like I was wasting so much time I could have been spending simply living my life. Enjoying every moment of what I thought I seeing the newsreader present a piece on the charity, calling out for people to apply for that gift.

My wedding to John back in 1996 in Las Vegas cost us all of $25. My bridal outfit consisted of a pair of denim shorts and a shirt I purchased from Target. John was wearing an acid washed t-shirt he had purchased earlier on our trip to Los Angeles. We had only known each other for four months. It was perfect at the time, but I had always wanted a 'real' wedding, looking like a real bride. When I found out we'd been chosen as the lucky couple, John and I were thrilled and honoured to have been chosen.

I felt like I'd won the lottery with My Wedding Wish. The only other time I've won anything in my life was when my mum raffled off some yellow salt and pepper ceramic cats at a Highland dancing competition when I was a young Scottish dancer. Even then, Mum had bought the tickets on my behalf.

On 1 June 2015, I renewed my vows with John at Maddock Park on Ewen Maddock Dam in Glenview. The scenic setting was beautiful. Nathan was exempt from wearing a suit for the occasion and preferred shorts and a t-shirt. Comfort for him, another ASD trait, is a priority. I felt unworthy of all of the special treatment I received from Lynette and the My Wedding Wish team. They went above and beyond to plan the event, and link me up with hair and makeup, photography and just about everything we didn't worry about when we first tied the knot in Vegas. I felt overwhelmed with gratitude. *All of these people are bending over backwards to create something special for us.* It was truly a heartwarming experience.

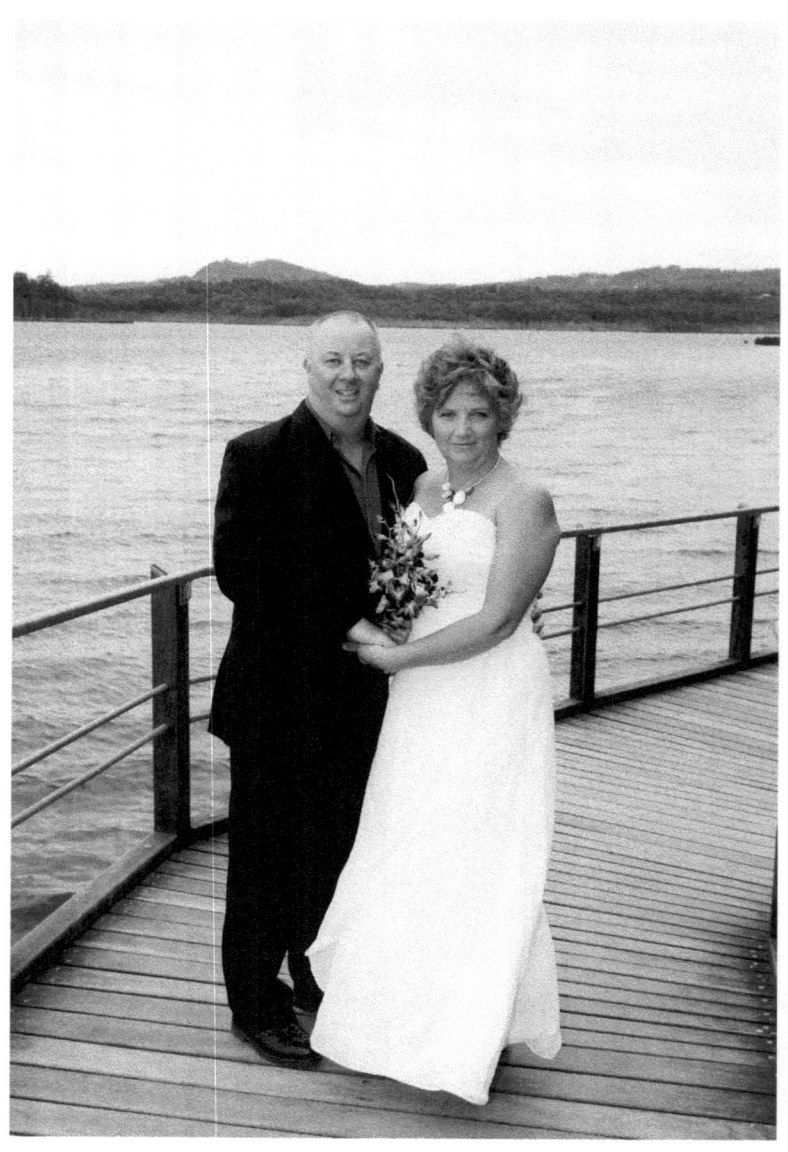

Our renewal of vows ceremony

We had an intimate ceremony with about thirty amazing people I had met since living on the Sunshine Coast. Friends also travelled up from Victoria and from Western Australia to celebrate with us. I treasure some deeply fond memories of that day, although I did miss having my parents and siblings there to celebrate with me.

I had a photo of our Vegas wedding blown up into a big poster and put it on display at our 'white wedding' on the Coast, and people marvelled at it. They said I hadn't changed a bit since I was twenty-nine. They were not very good at lying.

It was moving to see John connect with the importance of our ceremony. I remember him being much more emotional than me! Nathan was just excited that there was cake.

As beautiful as it all was, I wasn't able to fully escape my health predicament. As I was taking the cannabis oil, I was prone to dehydration and through all the goings-on, I hadn't drunk much water that day. Dry mouth, an effect of cannabis, and dehydration had made my breath smell. I was embarrassed as I imagined I was emanating a morning breath scent onto everyone who came up to me and congratulated me. I became extremely self-conscious. Luckily, no one else seemed to notice before I managed to track down some mints and temporarily fixed the situation.

As I write this, a part of me feels a little guilty that we were treated to all of this when I am still standing years later. I was one of the lucky ones who was able to cheat a terminal diagnosis, or at least somehow barter for an extension on my expiry date.

We left the party in a Kombi van convoy, in homage to John's love of the trusty Volkswagen. The following day, a few close friends and John, Nathan and I spent three nights on a houseboat soaking up the sights along the Noosa River. It was a mini honeymoon filled with laughter – one I will never forget.

My bestie and unlikely friends

September 2015

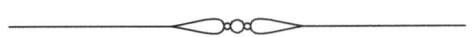

Just when I thought I had reached the bottom, the lowest of the lows, when I started chemo, I was told my best four-legged friend was riddled with cancer. I had begun to notice that Flea was becoming ill. At first, I didn't know what was wrong with her. When I took her to the vet, they were quick to pick up that her lymph nodes were enlarged throughout her body and they told me it was likely to be cancerous.

This was devastating news. My heart broke as I realised my beloved pup was going through a similar trauma to the one I was going through. Flea had been the one who had motivated me to get up every morning and to try my utmost to stay active, even if the walks were shorter and less frequent than they had been before I became ill.

Flea had been by my side for sixteen years. Each morning, at the same time, I heard her trotting down the hall, her feet tapping on the floorboards as she approached the bedroom.

Flea tucked her cold, wet nose under my elbow and lifted it up. This woke me every time. Sometimes I would hate it, especially on cold, dark winter mornings.

Still, I followed her lead and took her for a walk every morning, even if I was in a zombie-like state. Some mornings, if time permitted, we would go further away from home, and on the weekends, we did our big runs.

Random smells in the bushes along the footpath would catch her attention. She would dart across in front of me. I became aware of this possibly happening, as I had tripped once before, so I was always prepared to hurdle her. She kept me alert at all times. And literally on my toes.

When we arrived at our Mooloolah shed, where there were no fences as yet, Flea never tried to run away. She was always near my feet and followed me everywhere. When I was hanging washing, she would lie on the concrete in the sun and watch me from no more than three metres away. One day we forgot to lock her in the shed while we went out for the day. I didn't even realise we had left her outside until we arrived home to find her lying on the doormat out the front of the shed. When she saw us come home, she trotted up to the car, wagging her tail to greet us all. She couldn't understand the commotion and extra cuddles she was receiving that afternoon. We were so relieved she didn't run away. The opportunity was there but she never took it. She was such a special girl.

As Flea got a little older, I didn't run as far with her. She was tiring sooner. I thought it best not to take her on my runs and just go for walks around the block each day. On some occasions,

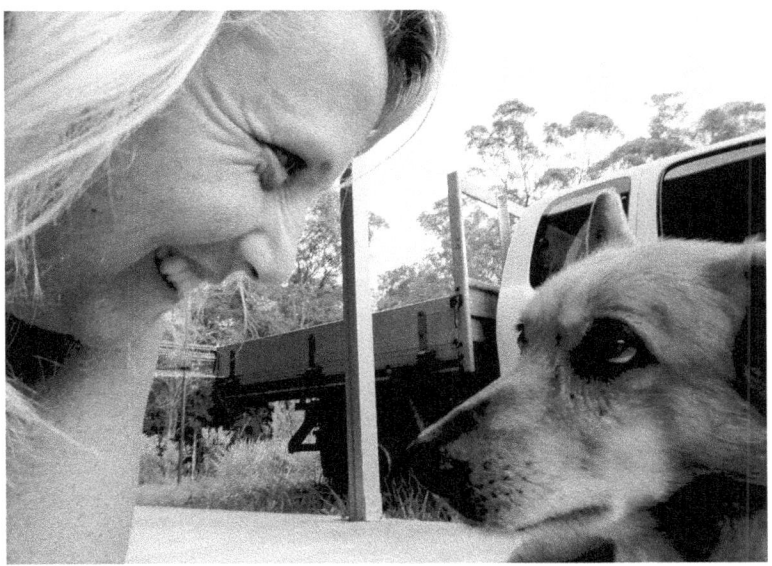

Flea gave me motivation – right up to the end of her life

she just stopped running and sat on the path. One day I had to carry her a little of the way.

I took Flea for her yearly check-up and asked the vet about a mass that had appeared near her neck. He mentioned she was starting to get arthritis. Her sight was also deteriorating, which would cause her to trip over things.

Flea and I continued to walk around the block each morning. She knew the route easily and when she was off the lead, she would run a little bit further ahead and then stop. She turned around, looked at me and waited as if to say, "Hurry up!"

But over time, another lump formed near her leg, making it hard for her to walk. He said if Flea had surgery, it would not be of benefit to her because of her age.

When I started chemotherapy, Flea was never far from me. She followed me into different rooms in the house. I felt as if I had become her guide and we were each other's support person.

As my energy returned, Flea's began to wane, and on hot days, I carried her to our pool and gently lowered her into the water with me. It was good for her joints and she seemed to warm to the idea after a while. This was the only time she never came to me. She preferred to swim to the steps and clamber out.

Soon, Flea was in such discomfort she couldn't go to the toilet. When I took her to the vet, he said the cancer had advanced.

We asked for the vet to make a house call in the afternoon and we had Flea put to sleep while she lay on my lap. We buried her near the clothesline so she can still watch me hang out the washing.

My runs were never the same without Flea and I felt a lot of grief as I picked up the pace while training for the next Foreshore Fun Run, which I had entered every year since moving to the Sunshine Coast. It became a drive to keep me going. I participated in the fun run two months before my kidney surgery and continued every year. I wasn't interested in the times I ran it in but just felt I needed to be there and give it a go. Something to look forward to. A goal.

I continued to run as best as I could with a limited supply of energy and on inconsistent days. Some days I woke up feeling on top of the world. On others, it was a mission simply to drag myself out of bed.

Throughout my journey I have had to deal with some awful situations, times when I felt vulnerable and extremely sad and down, thinking that life had already thrown enough punches. How can life be so cruel to add more crap? It is amazing how people who you thought were true friends sometimes end up being nothing of the sort. I started questioning myself. I was feeling so lost. Maybe I had caused some of the fractures in some of the friendships. But true friends, lasting friends, and some professional counselling helped me understand. And put me back on track.

I was able to conquer another obstacle and it made me a much stronger person. Friendships that had been a pillar of strength for me during my early days of battling cancer were finished. It really broke my heart.

I have drawn on this experience in my life. It has been a stepping stone. A challenge. Part of my journey. I actually feel that it was meant to be. I wrote heartfelt, unsent letters. It was a form of emotional release. This other 'cancer' of the heart has now been removed and I have closure. I have moved forward and it has given me the opportunity to meet beautiful people and develop new interests that enrich my soul.

I came to realise that people arrive in your life for different reasons. Some arrive and never leave – they are your kindred spirits and the ones who are with you through thick and thin. Some come and go quite quickly but can have an impact on

> *I was able to conquer another obstacle and it made me a much stronger person.*

your world – for better or worse – in the short time they are there. Others come into your life purely to teach you a lesson of some kind or may simply hang around in the background as comforting constants without ever being a prominent force in your life.

Unwelcome returns

November 2015

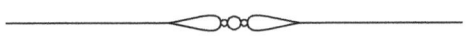

We had planned to head over to Perth the following month to see a couple of friends from school in Port Hedland, but my world came crashing down once more when a regular CT scan, which I'd had every three months since my kidney was removed, revealed a mass growing in my groin. A PET scan showed it was indeed another tumour. The oncologist confirmed I would need to treat this tumour with radiation and allowed me to go ahead with our scheduled visit to Western Australia before we began.

I was devastated and immediately thought all of my efforts with the cannabis oil had been for nought. I was truly in disbelief. I had never fully believed the oil would be a cure, but I had only been taking it for just over twelve months at that stage and I guess I had hoped it would give me more time. I was twenty-six months post kidney removal surgery, and I had started to feel like my 'bonus level' had kicked in as I had outlived the initial two-year prognosis.

This tumour, however, was a real kick in the teeth and I felt so low. Before this scan, my energy levels were starting to return. I was getting active again and was out enjoying the gardens I had created over the years as often as I could. My mind was in a positive state up till then, even if I always knew deep down I wasn't fully out of the woods.

I debated in my mind whether I should tell my medical team about my use of cannabis oil. I was unsure whether it would open me up to being reported to the police or if they would be receptive and supportive of my choice. Eventually, I decided to tell my oncologist.

The oncologist looked at me with a serious face and simply said, "It sounds a bit recreational to me." I shrugged my shoulders, relieved there were no repercussions but also slightly deflated that he didn't see the value in what I was doing to help myself. His opinion of medical cannabis was that it was simply something that was all the rage now.

> *I debated in my mind whether I should tell my medical team about my use of cannabis oil.*

However, he pointed out something interesting to me in one consultation and it lifted my spirits when I was feeling so low and powerless because the cancer had returned to the iliacus (near the groin) only four months after my course of chemotherapy had finished. He told me this: "If you were going to get cancer again after it was in your left kidney, it would have been in your liver, bones or your brain. Usually what happens is it will infect everything along the way as it moves through your lymphatic system in your body." The cancer was in the iliacus on the right-hand side, below the remaining kidney.

When I was first diagnosed with collecting duct carcinoma, the entire left kidney was removed. The second tumour appeared above my groin, on the right side of my body. A daily course of radiation treatment was performed over three months. It appeared to disappear but left a mass of unseen scar tissue. I commenced taking the 'bombardment of cannabis oil', also known as titration,[48] four months after the second tumour was discovered. This didn't mean a thing to me at first, but then the realisation came that perhaps my insistence on taking my daily cannabis oil was what had stopped the continuous spread of the cancer cells and limited the areas of the body they infected.

The timing was all wrong according to the medical book. This is not the way cancer usually acts. I think you can generally tell if your doctor is going to be judgemental or not. Throughout my healing journey, I felt some oncologists/specialists would have been more open-minded and accepting of medical cannabis if it was legal at the time. But I chose never to bring it up with a medical professional again – not until medicinal cannabis was eventually legalised in Australia.

> *I chose never to bring it up with a medical professional again.*

I just don't like people shutting you down when you talk about it and I think that's probably stopping a lot of people who qualify for prescriptions for medicinal cannabis from reaching out and asking for help. They might know their doctor is old-fashioned or might look down on them for even suggesting such a thing. We still have a long way to go to remove the stigma around accessing this medicine in Australia. For those who have come up against dismissal, I would encourage getting a second opinion. Always ask questions. Become educated. Know your subject.

> *Always ask questions. Become educated.*

Releasing this book is the most open I've ever been with anyone about my use of medical cannabis oil. It was never something I shouted from the rooftops, for obvious reasons. The few close friends I did tell were accepting of it and were happy to keep my secret for me. But I have more confidence now to start conversations with people whom I think it might help. I was talking to a colleague at work one day when she mentioned one of her relatives was sick from cancer treatment and I suggested they try cannabis oil. It's about making people aware it is an option so they can do their own research and decide for themselves. The publicity around medical cannabis hasn't been very open. I feel a lot of people are still in the dark about how it is now accessible. The stigma is still there. Newsreaders who report on 'the war on drugs' probably don't realise the fact that the government allows exactly the same plant to be grown... of course, it's in a 'controlled environment' and it's 'medicinal'.

Another tumour had started growing very close to the last one. My right thigh had developed a nodule the size of a fifty-cent piece. Another biopsy was taken and my suspicions were again confirmed. I started radiation on the area of the third tumour in November 2015 to reduce the chance of any cancerous cells increasing and reproducing. I thought, *At least this will kill the tumour and I'll be cancer-free once again.* It seemed implausible that I wouldn't be able to tackle this as I had the previous two tumours. There was, however, a tiny voice that sometimes piped up in the middle of the night, *But what if it doesn't work?* I tried my best to suppress that voice as much as I could. I didn't want it to gain enough power to make me lose hope. On 1 December 2015, the second round of radiation on my third tumour was completed.

By early June 2016, I began to feel some niggling pains in my upper abdomen. Ordinarily, I would have just brushed something like this off as it wasn't excruciating by any stretch of the imagination. But since my cancer diagnosis, there was a certain level of cautiousness that I brought to my body and I was more dialled in to things that were out of the ordinary. Of course, there was a little part of me that thought, *Maybe the cancer is back.* The long and short of it was that I wasn't about to take any chances and let it go unchecked.

I went to visit my GP and he ordered an ultrasound to check the area. They discovered a series of small stones that were blocking the connection from my gallbladder to my small intestine. The gallbladder is a relatively underappreciated organ, but it is responsible for producing and holding the digestive fluids and releasing them into the small intestine. The blockage I had was causing inflammation of my gallbladder, giving me a condition known as cholecystitis.[49]

I didn't want it to gain enough power to make me lose hope.

I was immediately relieved and actually happy that cancer hadn't found its way into another organ, particularly because the liver is in the vicinity of the gallbladder and my research had shown that when kidney cancer patients experience metastasis, it commonly affects the liver. It feels strange to think I was relieved to be going under the knife for something other than cancer. The pain was intermittent and occurred if I exerted my core muscles, but the doctor recommended I go under the knife for a cholecystectomy – a fancy name for removing my gallbladder through keyhole surgery. On 30 June 2016, I had another organ removed from my body. During the post-op debrief, the surgeon took me by surprise when he announced I had somewhat different anatomy.

I had somewhat different anatomy.

I already felt like my body was pretty botched by the whole cancer situation, but he mentioned that he got a surprise when he went in to remove my gallbladder because it was actually located in the reverse position to 'normal' people. He was a highly experienced surgeon but said that, with the arteries and veins running alongside the gallbladder, he had to double-check everything before he made any cuts to be sure he didn't cut the wrong bits. Given that it was keyhole surgery, my recovery time was fairly speedy and I was back on my feet in no time.

The lead-up to each scan was tense as the what-ifs played out in my mind. Luckily, the three CT scans I'd had following the rounds of radiation at the end of the previous year had come back clear and I was starting to breathe easier again. It was nearly twelve months since radiation treatment began on my thigh tumour and I allowed myself to think, *Maybe I have actually defeated cancer!*

I was scheduled for a CT scan in six weeks' time, but I had a gnawing feeling that something wasn't quite right. I decided to bring it forward by a month. This was the first time I had truly listened to my body and I am grateful that I had reached a point where I was prepared to stand up and become my own health advocate. I could have easily passed over this sense of something being off and trusted that it would be okay to wait until the five months prescribed by my specialist had passed before going for my next scan. But I chose to be proactive.

> *I was prepared to stand up and become my own health advocate.*

It was a good thing I did because the tumour on my thigh had come back. A few weeks later, a biopsy of the tumour showed the CDC had struck again. An MRI scan on my thigh in November 2016 showed the tumour was about three centimetres long, but it was contained and not wide-spread.

Thankfully, this was all my medical team needed to give me clearance to continue with a South Pacific cruise I had booked six months earlier. Fiji was absolutely beautiful. We sailed over on a cruise ship and had an internal cabin, which was a bit confined with the three of us in there. A couple of my friends came along, which was fun. I did get tired a lot but was happy John and Nathan could go and do their own thing if I needed to rest.

After my return from holidays, I was shocked to find the tumour had grown another four centimetres in just ten days. It was, however, encased inside the muscle in my thigh, almost like a sausage in one of my adductor muscles. Nothing around it was affected. Something must have stopped it spreading, but they couldn't give me a definite explanation of what it could have been. I believe it was the cannabis oil doing its thing.

> *The tumour had grown another four centimetres in just ten days.*

Given the rapid nature of the growth, there was no messing around with it. On 16 December 2016, I had the tumour, along with the three abductor muscles which had surrounded it, removed from my right thigh. This is called a compartectomy. I quickly found the little things you need to do every day become big tasks when you've had surgery on your thigh. I remember when I tried to put my shoes on so I could walk around the block. Nathan was in bed and John had already gone to work, so I leaned over to pull a shoe over my heel and I ripped a few of the stitches in my leg. I was so frustrated not to be able to do the normal daily things I used to be able to do very easily.

A drain was inserted into my leg, which became a pain in the arse. It started coming out at one stage. Of course, these things happen only on public holidays. I went to my nearest hospital to have it fixed and they wouldn't touch it. This was because they had not inserted it in the first place. I was more than capable of adjusting it myself, given my training as a nurse, but they refused to let me know how far down my leg the drain was, so

I had nothing to work with. I was advised I had to go down to Brisbane where I'd had it inserted because the specialty suites at my local hospital were closed for Christmas. I managed to get my friends who were up on holiday to drive me down to Brisbane. The most frustrating thing was that it was a ninety-minute drive and it took them all of two seconds to fix it for me!

Part of my healing was that I had to wear a compression stocking, as I was developing lymphedema from the radiation and removal of lymph nodes a year earlier.[50] Swelling due to build-up of lymph fluid in the body is a common side effect. Lymph nodes act like a drain and if they get clogged, the fluid cannot drain away. When I was running, the only sign that something was not quite right was that my foot felt tired, floppy and numb. I was told I would have to wear the compression stocking for the rest of my life, which really upset me. Running was also to be a thing of the past, according to the surgeon.

I diligently measured my leg each night and kept up my appointments at the lymphatic clinic. The staff were so helpful there. Measurements of my leg were taken to keep tabs on the fluid build-up. One amazing day, I went into the clinic and the nurse assisting me smiled and said, "You don't need to come back anymore. The fluid is not staying around your ankle. Your lymphatics have built a new pathway back." It had never been mentioned to me that this could occur. I resigned myself initially that a compression

> *The nurse assisting me smiled and said, "You don't need to come back anymore."*

stocking would now be a part of my life, so I purchased three. They were expensive. They now sit in my wardrobe as another reminder of how far I have come and how the professionals do not necessarily know everything. My ankles were meant to be swelling, but they weren't. These new pathways had formed because I was active throughout the whole process.

As hard as it was some days to get out of bed and do any form of exercise, I kept pushing through. When I was undergoing chemo, there were days when I couldn't even make it up the stairs outside my house. But the fact I have been able to avoid wearing compression stockings despite having lymphedema shows how important it is to stay physically active.

At that stage, I was on a daily cannabis oil maintenance dose of two drops, taken as a suppository once a day. It is recommended as being one drop a day, but the consistency was so thick that I figured one drop would be hemp seed oil, which is used as a carrier oil, and the other pure, whole-plant cannabis oil.

Instead of taking drops under the tongue, I had moved on to suppositories. The reason for this was two-fold. My frenulum didn't have the swelling reaction which occurred at first and it had less of an effect on my cognitive abilities when I took the dose that way. I also felt the cannabis was going to internal parts of my body where it was needed more. All the tumours developed in my lower torso, so having the oil administered this way made more sense to me. I reasoned that if I took it orally, stomach acid would eliminate much of the important components that cannabis contained. I found an online health food store that sold vegetable capsules and bought a stack of them. I was able to take my cannabis oil supply and add the appropriate number of drops to each capsule with hemp seed oil as a carrier and keep them stored until needed.

We had managed to pack a fair bit of holiday memory-making time into the past few years, so we moved into a more settled stage of being at home and working on things to improve our little piece of paradise. I was slowly starting to build my capacity to get everything done around the home each day. When I'd first started chemotherapy, simply looking at the to-do list would make me feel physically sick because I knew it wouldn't all get done.

I was still working in the mindset of 'there's no time to waste', and the thought of leaving anything, no matter how trivial, incomplete or untouched sent me into a spin. It took me a while to navigate that mindset and allow myself to sink into the fact that I wouldn't have the physical stamina to complete everything in a day that I would usually have done before the surgery and treatment. Once I allowed myself the time to heal and to leave things for a few days, I began to relax a lot more into everyday home life.

I began to relax a lot more into everyday home life.

To this day, I feel like I'm not 100% how I used to be pre-operation. I used to be able to get up and have a running list of what needed to be done, where Nathan and I needed to be, and when I needed to work. I could juggle it all and not feel fatigued or confused about it. I find that I still struggle to sort mathematical equations in my head, like trying to work out quantities and transferring millimetres to centimetres quickly. It used to be instant with me, but now I have to concentrate to have any hope of working it out. I'm not sure what the cause of this is but it's my new reality.

I seemed to be more alert in the morning so would get up early to start the day and exercise if I was up to it. John used to get pissed off with me because I'd fall asleep in the recliner at 7pm. He used to blame the cannabis oil, but it really was the fact I would have been awake since 5.30am because I couldn't sleep and was ready to start my day.

As with most people, half-yearly dental visits are still a part of my life. Each time I attended my appointment my dentist cleaned my teeth and sent me on my way. I was happy no work needed to be done and bragged to John when I got home. At the time I didn't realise that my dentist didn't want me to be wasting my money on dentistry due to my terminal diagnosis. Making memories and having fun holidays was money to a worthwhile cause. Then he made a confession. After I had been in the clear with cancer for some time, he summoned up the courage to tell me that I actually needed six more crowns! I thought this was amusing and very thoughtful of him that he didn't want to burden me with extra dental work and expense while I was undergoing treatments, surgeries and everything else.

Insomnia was unwelcome, but with me it was frequent. Usually, it was brought on by overthinking about the previous day's events or forward-thinking about what I've got to do. I'm the type of person who feels I am worthy when I am doing things. The result is I'm just continuously busy. John actually asked me the other day, "What are we going to do when we run out of things to do?" I said, "Are you kidding me? Once you've done them all, it's like painting the Harbour Bridge, isn't it? You've got to go back and start again!"

I can get overwhelmed with all the 'stuff' and sometimes wish we didn't take on so much with our property. Being owner-builders and having things to constantly work on around the property can be mentally fatiguing at the best of times. But I now realise I wouldn't want it any other way. The end result is the house of our dreams, just the way we wanted it. I realised that simply breaking each day down into smaller tasks and being okay with not having a completely full plate all the time was the only way forward.

> *I can get overwhelmed with all the 'stuff'.*

The lethargy I felt was one of my biggest challenges. It's hard to tell if it was the leftover effects of the chemotherapy or the cannabis oil, or a combination of the two. Research shows some chemo side effects only affect your body in the hours after a treatment, while others can linger for years or remain with you always.[51] Having my four-legged accountability partner in Flea and then Angus, my current fur baby, who joined our family in August 2017, really helped me to fight off lethargy most days and avoid becoming a couch potato. This has helped me immensely in the long run.

I never considered stopping the cannabis oil to try to get rid of the lethargy. The only time I truly felt the cannabis was responsible for 100% of the lethargy was when I was at the peak of my bombardment treatment at forty drops a day. I admit I was in a different state for those days. Once I dropped back to the maintenance dose, I adjusted quickly and became more like myself.

Mental health roller coaster

To say I'd been through the wringer several times over is a bit of an understatement. To bounce between the joy of celebrating every clear CT scan and the devastation and uncertainty that comes whenever an anomaly is detected is not an easy lifestyle to live. The reality is, I don't feel 100% confident that I don't have cancer. I don't think you ever do. It's like a black cloud forever hanging over your head and you are wondering, *Is it going to show its ugly face again?*

Like anyone who is diagnosed with a terminal illness, I went through the stages of grief. I wouldn't say I experienced them in the lineal five-step stages you read about in some books. It came and went depending on where I was at in my journey at the time.

It's like a black cloud forever hanging over your head.

When I was studying for my nursing course, we had to complete an assignment in relation to the five stages of grief:

denial, anger, bargaining, depression and acceptance.[52] Usually these stages are after someone close in your life dies, but they can also apply to traumatic occurrences in life. I never believed I would be the one living these stages and coming to understand them so intimately. My grief journey started long before my cancer diagnosis with the death of my mother.

> *Cancer was not something I had planned on getting.*

Then, at the same time that I was dealing with my own emotions and stages of grief linked to receiving a terminal diagnosis of my own, I was trying to process the death of my father and the loss of love from my siblings. The death of a family member is traumatic, but the distancing of my three sisters was a lot harder to understand and accept. You could say this has been a rollercoaster of grief. I am not unique in this, I know. Everyone has experienced some form of loss in their lives.

My rollercoaster of emotion and grief looked like the following. It always helped me when I was able to receive confirmation from someone else that I wasn't messed up and the emotions I was feeling were perfectly normal.

1. Denial

When I first received the diagnosis of collecting duct carcinoma, denial was undoubtedly the first reaction I had. *It can't be true. I look after myself. I eat healthier now. I go to the doctor whenever something isn't right.* I am not one to get sick. Cancer was not something I had planned on getting. The whole reason for me to become healthy all those years ago was to not be a burden on the health system and on my family. I chose to be proactive. I chose to be the best I could possibly be. I left my awful self in Victoria. I had flipped sides from unhealthy to healthy. So why did this all happen? *It's just not fair.*

My sister's blasé attitude to all of it, telling me I was overreacting and had nothing to worry about, was a shock. To her, I was a hypochondriac. It was much easier to continue thinking all was well than to allow myself to think what it would mean for me if it wasn't.

When I first found out about my dad's health, he played it down so much that I was lulled into a sense of denial over how serious it actually was. It wasn't until I was called and told I had to say goodbye that I began to comprehend what was happening. I have regrets I couldn't do more at the time, but I also felt Dad would have totally understood my reasons for not being able to.

I was in denial about my siblings and I tried many times to reach out to them, only to face brick walls every time. I didn't want to believe that they were walking away when I really needed them the most. It was hard then. But now I have proven how strong a person I have become. I do not let it eat at me anymore. My siblings have denied Nathan the chance to meet his cousins. I openly talk to him about what they were like. In my own upbringing, my siblings and I did not know our cousins throughout our childhood because my parents did not like their

> *All the research I had to do, wasting precious time, could have been better spent.*

siblings. I would support Nathan should he try to seek out his cousins someday.

I have resentment about being denied cannabis oil from the beginning. While other countries around the world were miles ahead with everything to do with the subject, Australia was reinventing the wheel and running its own tests. The fluffing around may have been the reason my cancer had metastasised. All the research I had to do, wasting precious time, could have been better spent.

2. Anger

Once I realised this diagnosis was real, I had to learn to live with the outcome. *How am I going to move on from this? I don't deserve this! What did I do so wrong that I need to be punished in such a way?*

I knew I wasn't really fit and healthy until around 2003, when I decided to make a positive change in my lifestyle. Before that, I was suffering from sciatica, I was overweight and had smoked up until Nathan came into my life. I knew I had to kick the habit because I was entering into emphysema territory. I knew I was doing all the wrong things and was on a path to killing myself through bad choices.

But I had stopped all of it. I stopped smoking. I stopped being sedentary. I stopped working in a job environment I hated. I started to move and get excited about exercise and a healthy lifestyle. I was doing everything right and had been for almost a decade when the cancer was discovered. I felt like I was finally living. I became angry when I got diagnosed with cancer.

I set off on a mission to find out how this could have happened. *Who could I blame? Why did this happen to me?*

Those three-letter words – 'who' and 'why' – consumed me for months as I tried desperately to link my cancer to *something*. I didn't have any of the usual risk factors nor did I fit the profile of a 'typical' CDC patient. It wasn't my current lifestyle but was it the cumulative effect of the years before? With both of my parents dying from different forms of cancer, was I genetically predisposed? Was the environment I had worked in part of the problem? Was it the asbestos in the machine guards at the factories I worked at? I quickly found out that even if I could tentatively link it to this, I had worked for a tobacco company and we were required to sign waivers to the effect that we couldn't sue in the future. The reality was, I was never able to pinpoint what caused it and this fuelled my anger at the unfairness of it all.

> *I knew I was doing all the wrong things and was on a path to killing myself through bad choices.*

There were many times when I felt helpless. It was all out of my control. Everyone reacts to this differently. My reaction was anger. I was also angry that it was so hard to find legitimate and trustworthy information for my treatment and healing journey. The amount of information out there was daunting and it was hard to separate the good stuff from the utter crap. There were so many websites that claimed cannabis oil was the miracle cure for cancer. I never believed that, but I wanted to find a middle ground. I came across a site called United in Compassion,[53] and was able to find a community of people as well as information I could rely on. This wasn't an easy find back then; however, I'd seen it mentioned in a newspaper article.

> How could they do this to their own blood?

I was angry my dad had chosen not to seek medical help for so long. He was the stereotypical stubborn male and refused to acknowledge anything was wrong with him, no matter how hard he struggled to breathe or how many aches and pains he was dealing with. With most cancers, the chances of a good prognosis are much better the earlier it is detected. But because Dad put off doing anything about his health until he was in a dire state, early intervention was not possible.

My sisters' actions also angered me. *How could they do this to their own blood?* There has always been an element of anger simmering beneath my sadness. In the instance of my siblings, I could not understand why they had chosen to stop all communication with me. Nathan's relationship with his cousins and aunties became void once the communication ceased.

I was still angry with the world for being the way it was at the time – not allowing me free and easy access to the natural medicine I needed for my recovery. Not enough is being done to inform people about this option available to them, even now. I still get people calling me and asking me about the subject because they don't know where to begin. Why isn't the subject broadly communicated on television and radio, and spoken about like the weather? This infuriates me. It's still so stigmatised.

3. Bargaining

The concept of karma was something I had always valued. Do good and good will be done to you. Be a crappy person and your life will become a bit less shiny. When I reached the bargaining stage of grief, I began to really sink into the idea that if I changed my behaviour and became a better person by doing more in my community, maybe it would be enough for me to survive. Maybe, something positive would happen to me and my life would be spared.

I know there are different ways that people bargain. I played this phase out by fundraising for a couple of charities and raising awareness for The Forgotten Cancers Project, an initiative of the Cancer Council.[54] With such a high percentage of cancers being classed as 'rare', it blew my mind that they did not receive nearly as much funding or support as breast, lung and prostate cancers, and I wanted to do what I could to lend my voice to the growing number of people who have very limited treatment options due to lack of funding and research for the less common cancers.

Doing good for others and paying it forward ... feels right to me.

When I found out Dad was dying, I flew straight down there to be with him. Even though I was in severe pain and was losing blood every time I went to the toilet, I couldn't bear the thought of not being able to say goodbye. I guess I hoped by showing up, I would be able to remind him of how much he was loved.

As my siblings were beginning to pull away and I attempted contact with each of them with a heartfelt message, it fell on deaf ears. I never heard back from any of them.

I sometimes feel I am still in this phase of bargaining to some extent. I seem to value people more. I want to help people more. I do it now because it lights me up and makes me happy. Doing good for others and paying it forward with these extra years I have been able to live feels right to me. I can do this each day when I walk through the doors of my workplace.

I'm not an angel or anything, but I do believe this whole terrible experience has made me a nicer person.

In some respects, I think turning to cannabis oil was a bit of bargaining. I felt like it was my last-ditch effort to give myself a chance at life. Despite the inner conflict of going ahead with something that was illegal at the time, I decided I was ready to deal with the consequences if it ever came to it. I was prepared to do anything and try everything within my power to survive.

> *I was prepared to do anything and try everything within my power to survive.*

The moment I started taking the oil, I felt better in my mind. Because back then, I knew the cancer was in my body and there was a potential that it would run rampant if I couldn't stop it in some way. The idea the oil could help to slow or stop the cancer from growing and spreading was all the hope I needed. It was really a no-brainer.

Writing this book is part of the bargaining stage, I guess. Helping others to learn what took me years to find out makes me feel I have done something to help someone. I needed to share my knowledge and inform. To leave the planet without sharing my story would be selfish of me.

4. Depression

There were days when I wondered why I was still breathing. The mammoth weight of a terminal diagnosis can make you wonder sometimes why the inevitable is delayed. The uncertainty around whether you will make it to the end of the timeframe the doctors have given you can play tricks on your mind. On some days, particularly shortly after I received my cancer diagnosis, it was hard to manage the dark thoughts that crept in without warning. Deep down, I am still sad this has happened to me. The panic attacks that wake me during the night are real.

I still have down days, because this cancer burden is always with me, but those

I had always been a mostly positive person.

days are not as bad as they were to begin with. I had always been a mostly positive person, someone who tried to find the bright side of things all the time. But my health journey rattled me, to say the least. My foundations were shaken and there were times when I struggled to find level ground.

After the loss of my father and then the loss of love from my siblings, I reached a point of depression which I had not seen since I was in my early twenties. In my sadness, I left my home and set off to walk to Maleny, which would take more than three hours on foot from my home in the Mooloolah Valley. It was the middle of summer, with the temperature at thirty-five degrees, and I chose not to take a water bottle with me. The first part of my journey was a steep gravel incline along Brandenburg Road, where cars would have little to no visibility for pedestrians along the winding track. None of that was of concern to me. This was my cry for help.

I was hoping I would dehydrate and melt into the earth without a sign.

Literally, I was hoping I would dehydrate and melt into the earth without a sign, or that a car might speed the process up by hitting me. I was lost, angry and completely devastated by everything that had unfolded in my life.

I was severely dehydrated by the time I made it to Maleny but I was alive. I dragged my feet into a shop and asked to use the phone. I hadn't taken mine with me. I didn't think I'd need it where I was planning to go. I called John and he came to pick me up. Concern was etched on his face when he pulled up to collect me. "What's wrong? Why would you do something like that?" I understand why he didn't get it. He has never had to live inside my head. I still find it hard to articulate to him what drove me to act that way. Sometimes, depression is impossible to put into words.

The loss of my dad and the fact that his funeral was being held as I was being wheeled in for surgery was an awful combination. I was deeply depressed that I wasn't able to be there with my family at that time. But as it turns out, 'family' is just a word.

'Family' is just a word.

The depression came in waves. There was never really one trigger; it largely rested on the frame of mind I would wake up with that day. Sometimes I was too tired to feel anything. Other days I felt like my old, happy self. Then there were days when my mind was abuzz with random thoughts and anxiety about my future mixed with regrets from my past.

I had another bout of depression during our family trip to Tasmania. This one, however, gripped my body with the ferocity of an explosion. Everything I had endured seemed to come to a head and I raced out of the motorhome, grabbed a stick and dug it into my arm and dragged it towards my elbow, which left an open abrasion about 15cm long. I didn't do it to kill myself; I was just so angry and frustrated, I had to do something. I had to *feel* something because that whole day, all I'd experienced was numbness.

Depression wasn't something that was new for me from 2013 onwards. I think I had already accepted it as part of my life. Prior to my cancer diagnosis, my twenties were the worst time of my life because I felt I was always alone. I am so pleased depression is more understood and spoken about now, although there is still a way to go. There are so many organisations around that can help, and accessing them doesn't have the stigma it once did. Whereas, when I was growing up, there was not much choice or assistance available.

My twenties were the worst time of my life.

But it's all in your mind, how you process things. For me, writing was a great outlet. I used to write a lot of poetry. I used to write a lot in diaries. I don't have any of those anymore, as I decided I never wanted to read them and re-live those feelings. Getting my Diploma of Professional Writing and Editing helped me immensely with documenting my journey in this book. I also found great joy in regular massages and running or walking.

5. Acceptance

Coming to terms with what the future may be is easier now that I understand my destiny, which is to be there for my family and to truly appreciate my son and my husband and all of the people who make my life wonderful. I allow myself to believe I will grow old and see my son with a family of his own.

Every scan I have brings a wave of emotion. There is always uncertainty about what is going on inside my body. Going from three-month scans to only having one every twelve months was positively scary. But since 2017, my scans have been clear. There is always a build-up of tension around scan time, also known as 'scanxiety', but there is overwhelming relief when they don't find anything and you attain NED (no evidence of disease).[55] I feel like I can live another twelve months. People talk about the joy of remission or being cancer-free, but I've never personally liked those words. The more time that passes, the happier and more contented with life I feel.

I had to accept this was my lot in life in order to be able to move forward and be the best person I can be. With a nursing qualification under my belt, I have found a career where I can give back daily. I still can bring happiness and a bit of laughter to people, like those oldies that I scoot around the dining room in their wheelchairs really fast or lend an ear to if they are lonely or want to have a friendly discussion. I accept that my profession has given me joy and keeps me positive.

Acceptance, for me, came with realising attitude plays a huge role in how I live my life. *If I don't help myself, no one else can.* My attitude has returned to one of gratitude and positivity. The power of having this type of mindset is well documented. International motivational speaker Tony Robbins defines its importance as being able to "make or break an individual. Your thoughts affect your actions. Your actions, in turn, translate into whether or not you succeed in your field, as well as influence the quality of your personal relationships and how you view the world at large."[56]

I never wanted to just quit. I had a choice to take back power. I keep my body fit and strong as much as I can to give it the best chance of defeating the cancer cells should I go through this again. I can choose to battle through fatigue and

> *I still can bring happiness and a bit of laughter to people.*

do what my body can at any given time – a few steps taken are much better than none at all.

Whenever I had a sense of moving forward, I felt better. This is where walking and exercise played a huge role for me. I am not yet back to running half marathons, but I am proud that I could get up and walk my usual route on the days when I was feeling like crap. Small steps taken daily will become giant leaps with consistency.

I found my mental health improved greatly when I was physically active. You can't change what's dished out to you. It is what it is. If I had a choice, I would have chosen a different cancer: one that was more common and had better recovery statistics. We are so lucky to have what we have now in the way of medical interventions, as well as finally having the approval of medical cannabis. I would have been dosing my mum and dad up if it were legal when they were sick. This gives me a kind of reassurance, a determination to survive. It takes time, sometimes years, to accept the loss of a loved one. With Dad's death, I had lost both of my parents to cancer and it was a hard pill to swallow. I now feel that both he and Mum are watching over me. There are times when I hear a whisper of Mum calling my name in the wind or something silly brings back a memory. It's comforting.

Small steps taken daily will become giant leaps with consistency.

It's quite funny when I think about how I could never keep any plants alive before moving to the Sunshine Coast. Since I began spending more time in my garden as a means of escapism and calming myself down, I have been able to channel Mum's green thumb. Planting new things and bringing them to life. Waiting for new growth to appear.

At the start of my journey, I couldn't see a clear future. I felt like it had been taken away from me the moment I got the diagnosis. Now I feel more comfortable with moving forward, with continuing to plan for the future. I have been lucky enough to receive five more years following my last tumour surgery, also known as remission, and am now ten years down the track after being told I would have around two years left to live.

I accept that my life will never be as it was before 2013, but I also know that what I have been through has made me stronger mentally than I ever would have become without this journey.

"Everything happens for a reason."

My reaction to that statement would have been very different depending on where I was at on my journey. I had always believed it to be true, but when I ventured into the anger stage of my grieving process, I didn't believe there was a reason. I felt victimised and powerless. Now that I have reached a stage of acceptance, I know everything we go through is there to teach us some form of lesson, to make us stronger in some way.

You get one chance at life. The crap I went through in my early working life taught me not to sell myself short and to find a career that lit me up and made me want to go to work every day.

> *I am now ten years down the track after being told I would have around two years left to live.*

> *I know everything we go through is there to teach us some form of lesson.*

My poor health taught me there was a better way to live and led me to a life-changing health move. The relationship breakdowns with friends and my family showed me not to waste time with toxic relationships and not to read too much into things.

I appreciate life so much more now because I have a very real understanding of the fact that you never know when your time is up. I am also very proactive about my health. I exercise and eat relatively well. I carry out body checks, looking for bumps, lumps, dimples, anything that has changed, and I monitor it all. I encourage every one of you reading this book to do the same. The World Health Organization says early detection of cancers greatly increases the chances for successful treatment.[57] Check your body and become your own best health advocate. If something doesn't feel right, ask your GP. If their response doesn't satisfy your worries, see another one! One thing I had to come to accept is that GPs, while incredibly knowledgeable and professional, are, at the end of the day, just humans too. They too can sometimes make mistakes.

I'm more in touch with how I feel now than I ever have been before. I'm also mentally stronger, because I feel like the brain has a lot to do with trying to get rid of cancer. What you do with your body and your thoughts means so much. Your negativity won't help you. You have to be positive. So, even if that's saying "Hello" to someone as you pass them in the street or having a little joke about something with some random person, it can be enough to lighten the mood in an instant. I do it all of the time. People must think I'm a real crazy sometimes. I just talk to strangers while I'm out and about. It has a double-whammy effect really. It makes me feel good and, you never know, you might be the only person who says "Hello" to that person for that entire day.

I get aches and pains in my body, like anyone my age does, and I have to stop that inner voice that squeals, *Maybe the cancer is back!* I have to not allow myself to think the worst. Usually the pain is gone in a day or two and I realise I have strained my body in some way – *bootcamp on Saturday caused that pain!* If it persists, I don't muck around anymore, it's straight off to the doctor I go.

Research shows that people who can implement effective coping strategies to deal with stress have lower levels of depression and anxiety and even reduce the symptoms they experience from cancer and its treatment.[58] It is so important to find what makes you feel better. I have seen a psychologist and gone down the counselling route, but I had to look around for the right fit. One psychologist I saw spent an entire session nodding her head and saying, "I understand… " I knew she *didn't* understand. Whereas other psychologists have been empathetic without trying to come across as understanding. I guess we all have our buttons and that was one that made me feel like that entire session was a waste of time.

> *Angus, my dog, helps with motivation and encourages me every morning.*

The outlets I used to feel better included writing, lymphatic drainage massages, and walking or running, depending on my fatigue levels.[59] I have built up a great relationship with my massage therapist and she sometimes doubles as a counsellor, as I speak with her whenever I am on her table.[60] But hands down the cheapest and best therapy of all for me is walking. Getting out in the fresh air and simply moving my body. Angus, my dog, helps with motivation and encourages me every morning as Flea used to.

At the end of the day, I am still breathing. The fact that I am alive gives me something to be grateful for every morning that I wake up. It might've gone the other way, but I don't dwell on that. I've been given this gift. I could be on dialysis. I could be in a box. Reminding myself of these simple truths is what allows me to stay positive.

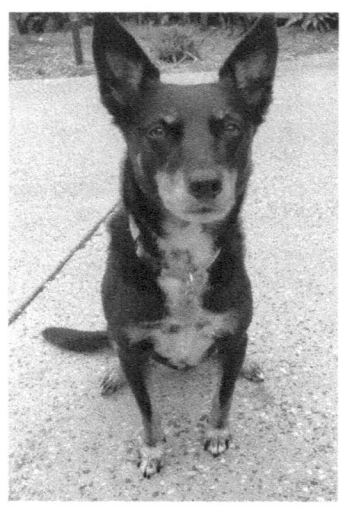

Our newest member of the family, Angus, who we got from the shelter in 2019

Smoking the stigma

Now that medical cannabis has been accepted in Australia, the stigma that is still associated with it needs to be removed.

For me, legalising medical cannabis was about freeing people from the fear I had endured since I began to take cannabis oil for my health. It's more than a little bit nerve-racking, because you know you are dealing with an illegal thing, but it was an essential thing for me and many others. To know there was a possibility people could access it without this fear, with open access to legitimate information and support, was the ultimate goal.

I was relieved when the laws were finally changed in Australia in 2016.

It was almost surreal in a sense because I had been fighting so hard to try and get it, writing to every Queensland Member of Parliament to draw attention to the issue

> **Now that medical cannabis has been accepted in Australia, the stigma that is still associated with it needs to be removed.**

in late 2015. Several replied with positive messages of comfort and support, but most return letters were computer-generated form letters. This made me feel so small and insignificant. I also got on board a formal petition, which was sponsored by then Buderim MP Steve Dickson. It attracted more than 12,000 signatures in around three weeks in favour of formal consideration of the cannabis treatment.[61]

> *This made me feel so small and insignificant.*

Medicinal cannabis was legalised under very strict guidelines and restrictions in Australia on 24 February 2016. In 2019, the Therapeutic Goods Administration (TGA),[62] which regulates medicinal cannabis in Australia, granted 25,182 applications from doctors to prescribe medicinal cannabis for a patient.[63] It is heartening to see this was more than a ten-fold increase from the previous year, but I believe there are so many people who are still afraid to ask about access to cannabis oil because of the stigma that surrounds it. However, the TGA has not accepted medical cannabis for use for shrinking tumours as other countries have, only for cancer-related nausea and reducing the effects of chemotherapy and cancer pain. What is cancer pain? I don't believe this can be singled out to one thing. Cancer pain is related to any pain that cancer is responsible for. So, anybody who has this type of pain can access medical cannabis.

While the government has legalised cannabis for certain patients, the wider community appears to still hold fast to the stereotypes introduced in the 1930s. Bring cannabis up at a social gathering and notice how many people get angry and say how someone they know is now addicted to hard stuff because of cannabis. It has been deemed a gateway drug by many who are swept up in the stigma that surrounds cannabis.

I was at a barbeque at a friend's house and the topic of cannabis came up shortly after medicinal cannabis had been legalised. I figured it would be much more socially acceptable to talk about it so mentioned I had used it on my healing journey. One of the ladies at the table became deeply offended because her son was schizophrenic. One of the leading arguments of the 'con' camp during the cannabis debate was that excessive cannabis use causes schizophrenia.

For the record, a Harvard Medical School article by Ann MacDonald published in 2020 examined the risk of teenagers who smoke marijuana developing psychosis later in life.[64] The study found there is only an *association* between smoking pot and developing psychosis or schizophrenia. "That's not the same thing as saying marijuana *causes* psychosis," MacDonald writes.

I am confused as to why the stigma is so strong.

I've come across many people who are anti-cannabis but have never smoked marijuana or tried cannabis oil. I guess it goes to show that we are so influenced by what wider society has to say. For many decades, the government has said it's bad, therefore it is. I am confused as to why the stigma is so strong. It's a natural plant, not something created in a laboratory, such as pharmaceutical medications, or in a dodgy backyard lab, yet it has been lumped into the same category as cocaine, heroin and ecstasy, which are all manufactured and cut with all kinds of impurities.

When you look at famous people from recent history, you may be surprised to see the calibre of the people who have admitted to smoking cannabis in their youth.

Former USA president Barack Obama admitted to recreationally smoking dope in high school but just didn't get caught.[65] He was able to maintain his highly intellectual capabilities as a thought leader and went on to become one of the country's greatest presidents.

Blockbuster megastar Will Smith and his family discussed being '420 friendly' (slang for someone who is accepting of those who smoke cannabis) in an episode of their Red Table Talk online series.[66] Forbes listed Smith as the tenth highest paid actor in 2019 with earnings of US$35 million.[67]

Microsoft co-founder Bill Gates publicly backed the 2012 referendum to legalise cannabis in Washington. A biography written by Stephen Manes states, "As for drugs – well, Gates was certainly not unusual there. Marijuana was the pharmaceutical of choice."[68]

Olivia Newton-John swore by medical cannabis to "help with my symptoms". She has also been quoted as saying it's a "healing plant" and "is something that should be available to everyone who is going through a chronic illness or pain".[69]

The cannabis community prefer the term therapeutic use to recreational use. Therapeutic is a term used to describe restoration of health and the treatment of illness,[70] while recreational relates to things people do in their spare time.[71] Many people in the cannabis community who use it recreationally are doing it to relieve their pain, not to party.

Research has found the negative image of 'potheads' smoking joints, which is reinforced by film and television to this day, influences public opinion that cannabis is bad for you.[72] However, a study by Bottorff and colleagues looked into the reasons why sick patients have turned to cannabis. The twenty-three individuals studied had various medical conditions including HIV, fibromyalgia, arthritis, anxiety/mood disorders, cancer, epilepsy and chronic pain. Their perception of cannabis was very different, with 100% of them describing it purely as life-preserving or a means of self-management for their conditions.[73]

According to the TGA, some of the approved applications for prescriptions for medical cannabis in Australia include:

- Nausea and vomiting from chemotherapy
- Severe childhood epilepsy
- Palliative care
- Cancer pain
- Neuropathic pain
- Spasticity from neurological conditions such as Multiple Sclerosis
- Anorexia and wasting from a chronic illness (like cancer).[74]

The path Australia walked to reach a place where medicinal cannabis was legalised was an interesting one. Before 24 February 2016, cannabis was a Schedule Nine drug in all

Australian states and territories, placing it in the same category as drugs like heroin and LSD.[75] Despite this, more than 300,000 Australians were reported as using it daily, largely for self-medicating for things like chronic pain, depression, arthritis, nausea and weight loss. Or people like me who were healing from cancer.

> *Medicinal cannabis is still a taboo topic.*

The latest debate around legalisation of medicinal cannabis sparked up in 2015. I was absolutely pro-legalisation, but I don't see myself as having played a large part in advocating for change. I supported organisations like the Medical Cannabis Users Association of Australia[76] and kept abreast of the topic as it trended in the media.

I was quite shocked at how quiet the debate appeared. There were the usual characters – politicians and medical professionals – presenting their point of view, but there were no massive protests or parades in the street. I firmly believe that's why there's still so much misunderstanding around it all to this day. Open and passionate debate would have had the benefit of educating the wider public about the pros and cons at the same time.

Because this didn't really happen, medicinal cannabis is still a taboo topic and not widely discussed. I believe there are so many people who could benefit from access to medicinal cannabis, but they are not sure how to access it or even if they are eligible to talk to their GP about obtaining it.

I can't wait for the day when it's a normal and acceptable thing to talk about. I hope this book is just one more step in that direction for our society. These should be casual conversations geared around providing people with other options for their health – not some loaded cloak and dagger conversation that could land you in jail. That should have dissolved the moment medical cannabis was legalised!

It frustrates me no end that the legalisation of medical cannabis in Australia has come with some of the strictest regulations around it. What this means is that pharmaceutically altered cannabis oil is now controlled by big pharma and they reap the financial rewards for a product that is, in essence, natural.

The price of medicinal cannabis products can vary greatly depending on what you are accessing and the quantity. The Victorian Department of Health lists costs from $50 to $1,000 per patient per week depending on the condition and prescribed dose.[77] Multiple Sclerosis Australia lists Sativex on their information sheets as a treatment option for patients. This is a mouth spray made up of the cannabinoids THC and CBD that can help with muscle stiffness that is common in people living with MS. The organisation says the cost of Sativex is approximately $745 for a six- to eight-week supply.[78]

It would not be in the government's best interest to allow people who are terminally ill to grow a couple of cannabis plants.

Imagine if cannabis oil were easier to obtain! I believe the pharmaceutical companies would go broke because cannabis can help with so many ailments. It would not be in the government's best interest to allow people who are terminally ill to grow a couple of cannabis plants and possibly live out their final days or years healing with a weed that grows freely in the back yard. They can't tax that.

In a perfect world, lives would be paramount above the dollar, but they are not. I could go on for a long time about this subject, but it's a whole other book or two... and this is just my opinion. When I was seeking a medical cannabis oil prescription, I rang a Sunshine Coast cannabis clinic in early 2021 and was informed the total fee would be $746 with the following breakdown:

- $299 for an initial consult
- $99 for an application to the TGA
- $149 for another appointment to collect the approval letter, prescription and a dosage diary
- $199 for a follow-up appointment

However, just recently (October 2022), the costs have dropped dramatically:

- $175 for an initial phone consult, which includes a follow-up call two weeks later by a nurse.

Some clinics offer a compassionate access program which offers a discount. My advice is to shop around.

The price for a 30ml bottle is between $175 and $199. And that can last around a month, maybe less. It's a lot of money if you are on a disability pension. At the time of writing, the prescription costs are not covered by Medicare or private health insurance.

I went to a Medical Cannabis Symposium in 2018 to see what I could learn about this big pharma approach to cannabis. I asked the founding director to explain what the difference was between the strains of cannabis they were using to produce the medicine and those that were accessible to the general public through previously illegal channels. He replied, "Nothing."

One of the businesses licensed to produce medical cannabis in Australia states on their website they have genetically superior strains that are backed by eleven years of scientific research in Israel, where the plants originated from.

In an article written by ABC journalist Jennifer Nichols, the founder of Medifarm Australia, Adam Benjamin, is quoted as saying, "If you look at the history books, scratch back to 1937, medical cannabis was the most widely prescribed medicine. American doctors, international doctors prescribed this. There is no surprise that the modern revolution in medical cannabis is gaining great traction."[79]

Back in 1937, medical cannabis was the most widely prescribed medicine.

When you look at America and its relationship with cannabis, it has really been a mixed bag. In the early 1600s, all settlers in the Jamestown colony were required to grow cannabis to help with supplies for the fibre used in textiles as well as the leaves and flowers for creation of cannabis-based medicines.[80]

The word marijuana didn't exist prior to 1910. It was simply known by its botanical name – cannabis. When the Great Depression arrived, the US federal government began treating cannabis as a foreign substance brought across the border by migrating Mexicans. With this move, the stigma around marijuana, then known as 'marihuana,' began to flourish. The swapping of the h with a j in the word is attributed to moves to further enhance the racial agenda against Mexicans.

The Marihuana Tax Act of 1937 was passed by American Congress and made the individual possession and sale of cannabis illegal, and any medicinal use became excessively expensive due to a fee system. Anyone who grew, bought, sold, imported, distributed or prescribed cannabis-based medicine had to pay a tax or face a fine or possible imprisonment for five years. In recent years, some US states have legalised medicinal or recreational use of cannabis.

In contrast, hemp seeds were not recorded in Australia until the arrival of the First Fleet in 1788. Early Australian governments supported the commercial growth of hemp for 150 years by gifting farmers land to grow the crop and providing financial incentives in the form of grants.[81]

Cannabis cigarettes, called Cigares De Joy, were widely available in Australia until the late 19th Century.[82] They were pushed as being able to provide immediate relief for asthma, cough, bronchitis, hay-fever, influenza and shortness of breath.

Cannabis was restricted to medicinal and scientific research purposes in 1925 when Australia became signatory to the Geneva Convention on Opium and Other Drugs. This grouped cannabis with morphine, cocaine and heroin.[83] Just three years later, Victoria passed legislation prohibiting cannabis use and other states followed suit over the next three decades.[84]

The shockwaves of the US movie *Reefer Madness*, created by director Louis Gasnier and producer George Hirliman, were felt in Australia in 1938 when cannabis was officially outlawed.[85] This is the first time Australians had heard the plant referred to as marijuana and the term was adopted here, along with the stigma that came with it.

Usage of cannabis peaked in the 1960s and 70s. During the latter decade, Royal Commissions and inquiries were held to combat the 'drug problem'.[86]

Influenced by the fact nine US states had decriminalised cannabis in 1977, New South Wales made an attempt to follow suit, but didn't succeed.[87] Australia has played with the idea since then, but time and time again has come up against the desire to continue the 'war on drugs' and cannabis remained firmly in the no-go zone as a result.

Interestingly, in 1994, the Australian National Task Force on Cannabis found the social harm of cannabis prohibition was greater than the harm from cannabis use.[88] By 2012, hemp seeds and other products became available in health food stores on the condition they were labelled with a warning the products were not for human consumption.

With hemp products available when I was on the lookout for products to help me, I could see how easily people were getting confused between what they could buy over the counter and the cannabis oil they actually needed but couldn't legally

The stigma around cannabis oil was huge.

> I was frustrated with the argument that it is a 'gateway drug'.

obtain. The stigma around cannabis oil was huge, even among people I connected with who were battling with the same rare cancer as me.

The real winds of change came when the Australian Government announced on 17 October 2015 that it would legalise the growing of cannabis for medicinal and scientific purposes. The Narcotic Drugs Act was amended on 24 February 2016 to allow for this, and medicinal cannabis was legalised on 1 November 2016. Almost a year later, Food Standards Australia New Zealand (FSANZ) made low THC hemp food legal for human consumption in Australia.[89]

Throughout this process, I began to feel a little more empowered to speak up. I guess I wanted people to shed their stereotypes about who a person accessing medical cannabis is. I was frustrated with the argument that it is a 'gateway drug'.

This could happen to any one of you. Don't judge me and other people accessing medicinal cannabis to ease their pain and suffering. And maybe, you might like to support the passing of these laws, because one day, you or someone you love might truly benefit from access to this medicine.

I truly hope, by starting conversations, I can create a small wave of change in my region so people might stop thinking of it as a taboo medicine. Back then, I was scared of raids and thought I might trigger one at my own home by speaking up.

I had heard stories of the police breaking into homes and taking oil, plants and equipment. Some of these people were producing it for compassionate reasons, not profit. I still worry about that now, even though I've got a script for the oil I have in my home. I never felt like a 'druggie'. I just felt like I was fighting a battle and I had to be focused on me, not any labels I might be slapped with in the process.

Unfortunately, there were other advocates for change who went too far, in my opinion. I guess any kind of debate has the tendency to polarise. There were those who wanted to keep cannabis locked out completely as a dangerous drug and there were others piping up that it was time to legalise it for any purpose and we should be free to smoke cannabis on the streets.

> *There were those who wanted to keep cannabis locked out completely.*

I attended a rally at a local library to find out more about what was being proposed and give my voice to the 'pro' crowd. But I was angry to leave the venue and walk through a cloud of cannabis smoke on my way to the car. All I could smell was dope. This small crowd of people decided to show their 'support' for the cause by lighting up joints in a public place. *What are you doing that for?* I screamed in my mind. *You're not helping the situation. You are only working to serve the stereotype we are working so hard to combat.*

At the time of writing, it is illegal to possess and use cannabis not medically prescribed in Australia. The only exception is the Australian Capital Territory (ACT). From 31 January 2020, the ACT legalised the possession and personal use of cannabis and allowed adults to cultivate up to two plants per person and four per household. Ironically, this is in breach of Commonwealth law.[90]

New South Wales has a compassionate use scheme for medicinal cannabis. According to the Centre for Medicinal Cannabis Research and Innovation, this gives police officers the opportunity to use their discretion to not charge adults with a terminal illness for possession of cannabis that has not been prescribed.[91] In my opinion, police officers are not doctors and should not be able to have the power of their 'own discretion'. Adults who have a legal document provided by their GP in the form of a script should feel free to take their medication 'as prescribed'.

It is an incredible difference to see what is available out there for people now. There are now Australian sites about medical cannabis that share research and information from credible sources. The information is a lot more open and it's easier to bust the myths that were prevalent while I was researching in a realm where it was still illegal to use it.

Laws are evolving so fast all the time, so much so, it would be wrong for me to write here what each state's laws are. This must be researched for yourself. Laws become outdated rapidly.

More research needs to be done around the effectiveness of using medical cannabis for the treatment of cancers like mine. At the moment, it is prescribed only to combat the effects of chemotherapy, not as a treatment for the cancer itself. This is because not a lot is known about the effect of cannabis on reducing cancerous tumours or reducing cancer cells in the body.

However, there is some promising work being done and I am optimistic about the future. Dr Matt Dunn of the University of Newcastle conducted laboratory tests over three years at the university and the Hunter Medical Research Institute and found a modified form of medicinal cannabis can kill or inhibit cancer cells without impacting the surrounding healthy cells.[92] The research, which was carried out in collaboration with the Australian Natural Therapeutics Group, produced a cannabis variety called Eve, which has less than 1% THC and has high levels of compound CBD. They tested it on leukaemia cells with great success.

This is the first bit of evidence I've seen that has allowed me to start to believe that maybe cannabis is more effective than I thought. I took it mainly because there might be a chance it might do something. I've never been 100% positive to say that yes it does cure cancer. I would never go there. But to have some research on it now is so heartening.

There will always be some people who fall through the cracks whenever regulations are in place. I know a man who was addicted to heroin in his youth. In a bid to get clean,

> *Medicinal cannabis can kill or inhibit cancer cells without impacting the surrounding healthy cells.*

he went on a methadone program. The program worked, but in later years he had a skydiving accident that left him with chronic pain. Even though chronic pain is one of the conditions that qualifies for access to medicinal cannabis, his misspent youth means he cannot access it. I believe, as we go on, there will be more and more people who will be excluded for this reason.

When I completed my nursing course, the mentality, even then, was 'doctors know best' and we have two or three generations of people walking this earth with that firm belief. When I listen to the views of the older patients I now work with, they are aghast at the thought of doing something other than what their doctor has told them to do or to consider taking anything other than what the doctor has prescribed for them. I've come to realise that *people will take handfuls of synthetic medication but not even entertain the idea of taking something natural.*

I know an older woman who was having trouble convincing the doctor she has been seeing for most of her adult life. "I want to access medicinal cannabis, but he just won't do it," she complained to me. She's been trying to twist his arm so she can take that instead of more synthetic medication but the answer is simpler than that – go to another doctor!

Whenever I was approached by people early in my cannabis oil days, I used to point people in the direction of Steve, the dealer, to help them with a supply. When I lost touch with him, I was really at a loss to be able to help people. Now I can say, "Talk to your GP and if your GP laughs at you or can't help, go to another GP."

> ## Prescription cannabis names
>
> The main names you will see used by Australian doctors when talking about medicinal cannabis vary greatly from the genus names already introduced in this book. Instead, you will find references to:[93]
>
> - **Nabiximols** – a TGA-registered medicine, under the tradename Sativex. It is a standardised extract of cannabis, containing roughly equal amounts of THC and CBD.
> - **Dronabinol** – a synthetic form of THC.
> - **Nabilone** – a cannabinoid created in the lab similar to THC, but with a chemically different structure.
> - **Ajulemic acid** – a cannabinoid created in the lab. It is similar to a breakdown product of THC but does not have psychoactive properties.

How to access medical cannabis – then and now

When medical cannabis was first legalised in Australia in 2016, the process to obtain a prescription for it was very involved, as outlined by the Australian Government Department of Health Therapeutic Goods Administration.[94]

Process to obtain medicinal cannabis in February 2016:

1. Medicinal cannabis can only be prescribed by a registered medical practitioner. This means your first port of call is your GP.

2. If your GP does not prescribe medicinal cannabis, you will need to find an Authorised Prescriber (AP) near you. Unfortunately, the TGA does not release a national list of APs, so you will need to ask around. This can be as simple as calling up GP clinics in your area and simply asking the question, "Do any of your doctors prescribe cannabis?" For links, see the Additional Resources page.

3. Before prescribing medical cannabis, the doctor will consider your family medical history as well as your own. Current medications and any issues with drug dependence and substance abuse become factors for eligibility as well.

4. The doctor will apply on the patient's behalf for approval to import and/or supply medicinal cannabis products through the Special Access Scheme (SAS Category A or B).

5. Approval is granted on a case-by-case basis.

6. If both state and TGA requirements are satisfied and the product is already in Australia, the product can be dispensed through a pharmacy or hospital organised by the prescribing doctor.

7. If the product is not yet authorised to be held in Australia, the doctor, or pharmacist or hospital on the doctor's behalf, may then need to obtain import permits from the Office of Drug Control.

Medicinal cannabis for personal use is certainly a lot easier to access now.

Process to obtain medicinal cannabis in 2023:

1. Your first port of call is your GP. Your doctor will print out your health summary and a referral form.

2. Select one of the many clinics from which you can now obtain medical cannabis. The choice is yours. There are also many different prices. It pays to understand different costs.

3. An appointment can be made in person (Medicare will subsidise this appointment) or via telehealth (not subsidised). The wait time can also vary considerably. One clinic had a waitlist of two months, the other was the next day by telehealth.

4. A doctor will call you or will see you in person. It will be discussed what form of medical cannabis will be prescribed at this time.

5. The script is faxed to the dispensary where your medicine is either picked up in person, which can be a distance to travel to some clinics, or can be posted to you for another fee. However, there are also risks with postage. If you ask the dispensary, you may be able to collect from one of their partners.

Epilogue – Moving on

2019

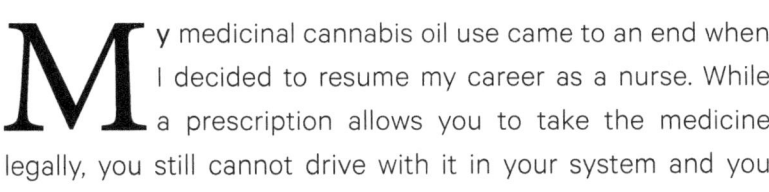

My medicinal cannabis oil use came to an end when I decided to resume my career as a nurse. While a prescription allows you to take the medicine legally, you still cannot drive with it in your system and you most certainly cannot care for patients.

It was an incredibly hard decision: one that took me months to make. Stopping the cannabis oil meant I was less tired and more alert, but my mind was hard to calm at times. *I'm dicing with death not taking my oil. What am I risking? Do I stay at home on cannabis oil to attempt to stave off cancer forever? Or do I re-enter society and hope the oil has done what it can for me already?*

For the five years prior, work hadn't even entered my mind. I was so focused on healing and beating cancer whenever it reared its ugly head. But I'd been fortunate enough to have five 'all clear' scans in a row and I was feeling more optimistic than ever before.

It was difficult to get back into the swing of working life again and fatigue was a factor in the early weeks. Late shifts were also a challenge to get through. But being amongst people every day, getting to know patients and being able to provide some comic relief from time to time has been the fuel that has kept me going since.

In the absence of cannabis oil, I have been taking a supplement containing MGN-3 arabinoxylan compound to help with my health. I started on the compound early in my cancer treatment after it was recommended to me by a naturopath to help with my immune levels. It has been reported to cause liver cancer cells to die and stop further cancer cells developing. It's also known as MGN-3 and is made from breaking down rice bran with enzymes from the Shitake mushroom.[95] At $490 for a month's supply, it's not the cheapest supplement around.

John and I did get out to Perth in 2018 and I was able to visit our friends Sharon and Dave from Port Hedland once more. I've known Sharon since I was fifteen and we shared a lot of our lives together even though we lived apart for many years. John, Nathan and I flew to Fremantle and stayed there for a couple of nights before heading off on a cruise to Singapore. We had a balcony room right next door to Sharon and Dave. We crossed the ocean and went touring together. John had a mate to drink at the bar with this time. Nathan was more social with Sharon and Dave, as they were a couple who were much more accepting of Nathan's traits than many are. The cruise was for

Sometimes things are just out of your control.

Epilogue – Moving on

twelve nights, but my family decided to stay an extra week to explore areas we didn't get to see while on the cruise. We then flew back to Brisbane.

I was unable to take my cannabis oil with me overseas, so I relied heavily on my MGN-3 arabinoxylan compound. I felt like at least I was still doing something proactive for my health.

When you're given a life expectancy of two years or even less, I think your whole world changes. Sometimes it's really painful to think about the family that I can't call family anymore. Sometimes things are just out of your control. I miss them all and think about them less.

I have gone from losing friendships with people I trusted to making new friends who would do anything for me and transitioned from someone who would never encourage taking recreational/therapeutic drugs to taking cannabis oil, and it changed my life along with my opinion on the matter.

I had taken cannabis for years and I remain positive that this gave me the best chance at life.

I've changed my point of view from looking at cannabis as a bad drug to now understanding and appreciating how it has been used for centuries for medical purposes and we are rediscovering this fact to assist with modern medicine practices. The two applications are so very different and the stigma around cannabis needs to change. I had taken cannabis for years and I remain positive that this gave me the best chance at life.

I have already shocked the doctors who said I would be dead in two years. Since then, I have been given a chance to celebrate many milestones. Even though I spent thousands of dollars on illegal cannabis oil – about $6,000 in all I think – it's a small price to pay if it has helped me to survive and to enjoy a good quality of life, to work, to travel, and to spend time with my loved ones.

> **Ask about cannabis if you think it may help you.**

Since my thigh surgery, I have persisted in my positive thinking and have pushed myself a little further every day to a point where I have become fit again and can enjoy running with Angus and the incredible feeling that comes with knowing I can do so without the muscle that was removed.

I would love to give Nathan cannabis oil to help him. He has been prescribed some by the doctor for his autism, but he is such a do-gooder – in the positive sense of the word – he refuses to take it. At least I have peace of mind, knowing that he and anyone else in this country can now access cannabis if they ever need to.

My wish is for people to take greater charge of their health and ask questions. Doctors are sometimes wrong and you know your own body better than anyone else. If you are not satisfied with what your doctor tells you, get another opinion. You are not betraying him or her. It's a business and, in some cases, you are just a consumer. Ask questions. Nothing is off limits. Ask about cannabis if you think it may help you.

Epilogue – Moving on

I have come to realise that some health professionals are not very good with people skills. My specialist showed a lack of compassion on an earlier visit, when he said in a roundabout way, "We all die of something, sometime." It's not the sort of statement you expect to hear, but I suppose he's immune to it. He tells people they are at death's door on a daily basis. I have come to realise an oncologist is not a psychologist and this highlights the importance of accessing support services to help you with your mental health during your treatment and healing process.

For me, massages, access to health services, asking for help, and running and walking were my 'things'.

Every single new pain or ache, I ask myself the question, *Is it cancer again?*

I feel absolutely privileged to have been given this extra time on earth.

I don't feel sick. Maybe that is the reason why I feel stuck in this place. The uncertainty of how the story will end has put my life in limbo. I once believed I had only two years left to live. That was years ago. I feel absolutely privileged to have been given this extra time on earth with my husband and son.

My body is recovering from the conventional treatments such as chemotherapy and radiation that took away the evil growing inside. Even though I have received 'all clear' scans since February 2017, there are physical scars and hot flushes to remind me of how lucky I have been. But I do feel happy and content. I will keep running. I'm not yet at the point of doing another half marathon, but my goal is to reach again that effortless running zone only a runner knows.

My hope is that by reading my story, you will find the strength you need to know there is the potential for a brighter future ahead for you too. Everyone's journey is unique; no person is exactly the same as another. I have no idea what it is about my situation that has seen me outlive a terminal stage four cancer diagnosis, but I hope some part of my journey inspires you and keeps you going.

If you or someone you know is in the battle of their lives, however low you may get, trust in yourself, help yourself, and live your days for yourself. This will reflect on the people around you for the rest of your life.

About the author

Allison McMaster was born in Melbourne, Victoria, Australia, to Scottish and New Zealand parents.

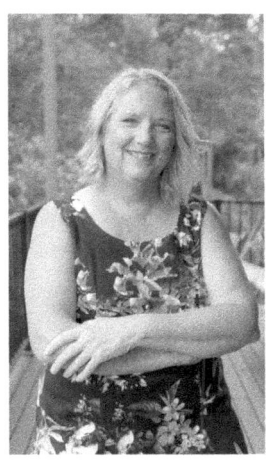

She lived her whole life in Victoria before moving to Queensland in 2009. During this time, she married and had a son and made many new friendships.

While working at a factory job in Melbourne in the 1980s, Allison decided to further her education and study to become a writer. She received her Diploma of Professional Writing and Editing in 1998.

The birth of her son Nathan and undiagnosed postnatal depression saw Allison's weight increase and career prospects seem out of reach until she met a personal trainer who managed to help.

Wanting to help others with fitness, Allison began to study once again and received her Diploma in Fitness and Personal Training.

The tough competition made it hard to find clients, so Allison hit the books again and did her Diploma in Nursing.

Armed with all this new knowledge and the devastating news of a cancer diagnosis, Allison decided to write her journey in this book.

Allison has been involved in stigmatised, illegal territory forbidden by the government to seek help and a possible cure.

Acknowledgements

This book is dedicated to my mother – the strongest person I know – who is supporting me mentally through this challenging time from the other side, wherever that may be.

There are also a fair few people who I still have the privilege of walking alongside on this earth.

My husband, John, has been the backbone of my journey and such a great support. He initially informed me of cannabis as a medicine, which has become the reason why I feel the need to share my journey. He has been my best friend for over twenty-five years and we can now look forward to many more in this bonus stage of my life.

Nathan, my son, has taught me how to be patient and how to value every extra day I have with him. He is my whole world and the reason I wake each day. I cannot describe here the joy and love I have for my little 'big' son.

Angus (and Flea) have motivated me each morning with sloppy kisses (licks) and motivation to go for 'walkies'.

Beautiful friends – they know who they are – who have been a part of my life pre- and post-cancer, and remain in my life to this day, have helped me through the really shitty times. I cannot thank them enough.

Additional resources

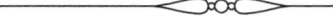

AlternaLeaf – alternaleaf.com.au

Canna Reviews Australia – cannareviewsau.co

Cann I Help – cannihelp.com.au

CDA Clinics – cdaclinics.com.au

Documentary *High as Mike*

Medical Cannabis Users Association of Australia – mcuainc.org.au

United in Compassion – unitedincompassion.com.au

References

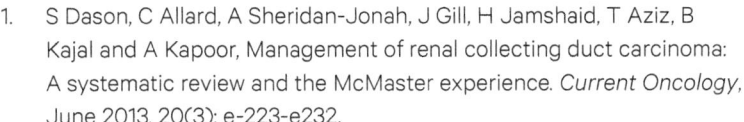

1. S Dason, C Allard, A Sheridan-Jonah, J Gill, H Jamshaid, T Aziz, B Kajal and A Kapoor, Management of renal collecting duct carcinoma: A systematic review and the McMaster experience. *Current Oncology*, June 2013, 20(3): e-223-e232.
2. Xiaoyuan Qian, Zhixian Wang, Jiaqiao Zhang, Qing Wang, Peng Zhou, Shaogang Wang, Bo Wang, Can Qian, Clinical Features and Prognostic Outcome of Renal Collecting Duct Carcinoma: 12 Cases from a Single Institution. *Cancer Management and Research*, 2020 12: 3589–3595.
3. Stages of Cancer. Cancer.Net. Retrieved from https://www.cancer.net/navigating-cancer-care/diagnosing-cancer/stages-cancer, September 21, 2020.
4. *What is rare or aggressive cancer?* MyCancer.com. Retrieved from https://www.mycancer.com/rare-or-aggressive-cancer/what-is-rare-aggressive-cancer/, September 20, 2020.
5. *Types of Cancer: Kidney Cancer.* Cancer Council. Retrieved from https://www.cancer.org.au/cancer-information/types-of-cancer/kidney-cancer, September 20, 2020.
6. Kyung A Kwon, Sung Yong Oh, Ho Young Kim, Hyo Song Kim, Ha Yong Lee, Tae Min Kim, Ho Yeong Lim, Na-Ri Lee, Hyo Jin Lee, Sook Hee Hong, Sun Young Rha, Clinical feature and treatment of collecting duct carcinoma of the kidney from the Korean Cancer Study Group, Genitourinary and Gynaecology Cancer Committee. *Cancer Research and Treatment*, April 2014, 46(2): 141–147.
7. *Types of Cancer: Kidney Cancer.* Cancer Council. Retrieved from https://www.cancer.org.au/cancer-information/types-of-cancer/kidney-cancer, September 20, 2020.

8. *Federal Election 2022 – Shifting the Dial on autism*. Australian Autism Alliance. Retrieved from https://australianautismalliance.org.au/shiftingthedialonautism/#:~:text=Australia's%20autistic%20population%20is%20estimated,of%20life%20than%20other%20Australians
9. *What is autism?* Autism Spectrum Australia. Retrieved on August 17, 2020 from https://www.autismspectrum.org.au/about-autism/what-is-autism
10. Leah Goulis, *The sad truth for parents of children with autism*. Kidspot.com.au, published July 19, 2017.
11. https://www.healthdirect.gov.au/sciatica
12. https://education.qld.gov.au/students/students-with-disability#who
13. https://www.pancare.org.au/managing-cancer-scanxiety/
14. *Types of Cancer: Prostate Cancer*, Cancer Council. Retrieved on August 25, 2020 from https://www.cancer.org.au/cancer-information/types-of-cancer/prostate-cancer
15. *Understanding Chemotherapy*, Cancer.Net. Retrieved on August 25, 2020 from https://www.cancer.net/navigating-cancer-care/how-cancer-treated/chemotherapy/understanding-chemotherapy
16. https://www.cancer.org.au/cancer-information/types-of-cancer/cancer-of-unknown-primary
17. *Treatment Methods: Chemotherapy*, Cancer Council. Retrieved on August 25, 2020 from https://www.cancer.org.au/cancer-information/treatment/chemotherapy
18. https://www.menopause.org.au/health-info/fact-sheets/early-menopause-chemotherapy-and-radiation-therapy
19. https://www.healthdirect.gov.au/medicines/brand/amt,72908011000036104/gemcitabine-dbl
20. https://www.healthdirect.gov.au/medicines/brand/amt,3785011000036102/cisplatin-dbl
21. *Cellulitis*, Mayo Clinic. Retrieved on August 25, 2020 from https://www.mayoclinic.org/diseases-conditions/cellulitis/symptoms-causes/syc-20370762

References

22. https://www.cancer.org.au/cancer-information/cancer-side-effects/peripheral-neuropathy
23. https://www.healthdirect.gov.au/magnetic-resonance-imaging-mri
24. Dying to Understand, https://www.dyingtounderstand.com/
25. *How Radiation Therapy Is Used to Treat Cancer,* American Cancer Society. Retrieved on August 25, 2020 from https://www.cancer.org/treatment/treatments-and-side-effects/treatment-types/radiation/basics.html
26. Dr Laura Martin, *Remission: What Does it Mean?* WebMD. November 11, 2018. Retrieved on September 17, 2020 from https://www.webmd.com/cancer/remission-what-does-it-mean
27. *Breast Cancer in Australia Statistics,* Australian Institute of Health and Welfare, Retrieved on September 1, 2020 from https://www.canceraustralia.gov.au/affected-cancer/cancer-types/breast-cancer/statistics
28. Xiaoyuan Qian et al., Clinical Features and Prognostic Outcome of Renal Collecting Duct Carcinoma.
29. https://www.rarecancers.org.au/
30. Aaron Cadena, *Hemp vs Marijuana: The Difference Explained.* September 11, 2018. Retrieved on September 15, 2020 from https://medium.com/cbd-origin/hemp-vs-marijuana-the-difference-explained-a837c51aa8f7
31. History.com editors, *Marijuana.* HISTORY, A&E Television Networks, October 10, 2019. Retrieved on September 15, 2020 from https://www.history.com/topics/crime/history-of-marijuana
32. *Reefer Madness* (1938). Public Domain Review. *Retrieved December 19, 2013.*
33. Cannabis Extraction: Learn about the various methods in which cannabis is extracted. MedicalJane. Retrieved September 8, 2020 from https://www.medicaljane.com/category/cannabis-classroom/extractions-methods/#types-of-cannabis-extracts
34. https://www.newcastle.edu.au/newsroom/featured/tests-show-potential-for-medicinal-cannabis-to-kill-cancer-cells

35. Crystal Raypole, *A Simple Guide to the Endocannabinoid System.* Medically reviewed by Alan Carter. Healthline, May 17, 2019. Retrieved August 25, 2020 from https://www.healthline.com/health/endocannabinoid-system
36. Kimberley Holland, *CBD vs THC: What's the Difference?* Medically reviewed by Eloise Theisen. Healthline, June 20, 2020. Retrieved August 25, 2020 from https://www.healthline.com/health/cbd-vs-thc
37. https://www.sciencedirect.com/science/article/pii/S0923753419390799
38. http://connections.edu.au/publicationhighlight/rates-characteristics-and-manner-cannabis-related-deaths-australia-2000-2018
39. Muhammad A Alsherbiny, Chun Guang Li, Medicinal Cannabis – Potential Drug Interactions, *Medicines* (Basel) 2019 Mar, 6(1): 3. Published online Dec 3, 2018. Retrieved July 3, 2021, from https://www.ncbi.nlm.nih.gov/pmc/articles/PMC6473892/
40. Eric Reed, *What are the side effects of CBD oil?* TheStreet, May 1, 2019. Retrieved September 28, 2020 from https://www.thestreet.com/lifestyle/what-are-the-side-effects-of-cbd-oil-14933788
41. Kimberly Holland, *Sativa vs Indica: What to Expect Across Cannabis Types and Strains.* Healthline, April 8, 2019. Retrieved from https://www.healthline.com/health/sativa-vs-indica#cannabis-strain-chart September 15, 2020.
42. https://shop.greenhouseseeds.nl/
43. Erica Cirino, *What You Need to Know About Herbal Tinctures.* Healthline, August 28, 2019. Retrieved September 15, 2020 from https://www.healthline.com/health/what-is-a-tincture
44. *Apoptosis,* National Human Genome Research Institute. Retrieved on July 3, 2021 from https://www.genome.gov/genetics-glossary/apoptosis
45. https://www.myweddingwish.org/
46. https://www.insider.com/guides/health/tincture
47. *Psychological Stress and Cancer.* National Cancer Institute. Retrieved on July 3, 2021 from https://www.cancer.gov/about-cancer/coping/feelings/stress-fact-sheet#how-does-psychological-stress-affect-people-who-have-cancer

References

48. https://cdaclinics.com.au/wp-content/uploads/Patient-e-book-journal-2021-FINAL-WEB-1.pdf
49. Cholecystitis. Mayo Clinic. Retrieved on July 5, 2021 from https://www.mayoclinic.org/diseases-conditions/cholecystitis/symptoms-causes/syc-20364867.
50. Phil Riches, *What is lymphedema?* Medical News Today, April 9, 2019. Retrieved September 9, 2020 from https://www.medicalnewstoday.com/articles/180919
51. *Late Side Effects of Chemotherapy.* Cancer Research UK. Retrieved September 21, 2020 from https://www.cancerresearchuk.org/about-cancer/cancer-in-general/treatment/chemotherapy/side-effects/late-effects \
52. Julie Axelrod, *The 5 Stages of Grief & Loss.* PsychCentral. July 8, 2020. Retrieved September 10, 2020 from https://psychcentral.com/lib/the-5-stages-of-loss-and-grief/
53. United in Compassion, https://unitedincompassion.com.au/
54. The Forgotten Cancers Project http://www.forgottencancers.com.au/
55. https://www.healthline.com/health/cancer/ned-cancer
56. Tony Robbins, *5 Strategies For Positive Thinking.* Retrieved September 14, 2020 from https://www.tonyrobbins.com/positive-thinking/
57. *Early Detection of Cancer.* World Health Organisation. Retrieved September 14, 2020 from https://www.who.int/cancer/detection/en/
58. *Psychological Stress and Cancer.* National Cancer Institute. Retrieved July 3, 2021 from https://www.cancer.gov/about-cancer/coping/feelings/stress-fact-sheet#how-does-psychological-stress-affect-people-who-have-cancer
59. Jamie Eske, *How to Perform a Lymphatic Drainage Massage.* Medical News Today, February 22, 2019.
60. https://rejuvenatemassage.com.au/
61. Richard Bruinsma, *Without cannabis oil "I'd be dead by now", says Sunshine Valley cancer patient. Sunshine Valley Gazette*, December 17, 2015.
62. https://www.tga.gov.au/products/unapproved-therapeutic-goods/medicinal-cannabis-hub

63. Tamika Seeto, *Medicinal Cannabis in Australia: Health Insurance.* Canstar, July 2, 2020. Retrieved September 15, 2020 from https://www.canstar.com.au/health-insurance/medicinal-marijuana-australia/

64. Ann MacDonald, *Teens who smoke pot at risk for later schizophrenia, psychosis.* Harvard Health Publishing, Harvard Medical School, March 6, 2020. Retrieved September 20, 2020 from https://www.health.harvard.edu/blog/teens-who-smoke-pot-at-risk-for-later-schizophrenia-psychosis-201103071676

65. Natalie Jennings, *The Choom Gang: President Obama's pot-smoking high school days details in Maraniss book.* The Washington Post, May 25, 2012.

66. *Will Smith's Emergency Family Meeting,* Red Table Talk. September 24, 2019. Retrieved September 14, 2020 from https://www.facebook.com/watch/?v=549708365774998

67. Madeline Berg, *The Highest Paid Actors 2019: Dwayne Johnson, Bradley Cooper and Chris Hemsworth.* Forbes, August 21, 2019.

68. Stephen Manes, *Gates: How Microsoft's Mogul Reinvented an Industry – And Made Himself the Richest Man in America.* Touchstone, 1994.

69. https://www.prevention.com/health/health-conditions/a39122778/olivia-newton-john-cannabis-cancer-treatment/

70. https://www.collinsdictionary.com/dictionary/english/therapeutic

71. https://www.collinsdictionary.com/dictionary/english/recreational

72. J Bottorff, L Bissell, J Balneaves, J Oliffe, J Capler, N Buxton, *Perceptions of cannabis as a stigmatized medicine: a qualitative descriptive study.* Harm Reduct J 2013, 10(2):1-10.

73. J Bottorff, L Bissell, L Balneaves, J Oliffe, H Kang, N Caple et al. *Health effects of using cannabis for therapeutic purposes: a gender analysis of users' perspectives.* Subst Use Misuse 2011, 46: 769–80.

74. Tamika Seeto, *Medicinal Cannabis in Australia: Health Insurance.* Canstar, July 2, 2020. Retrieved September 15, 2020 from https://www.canstar.com.au/health-insurance/medicinal-marijuana-australia/

75. Hamish R Smith, *Legalising Medical Cannabis in Australia.* Australian Medical Student Journal, July 24, 2013. Retrieved from https://www.amsj.org/archives/3022

References

76. https://www.mcuainc.org.au/
77. *Frequently asked questions about medicinal cannabis.* Health Victoria. Retrieved from https://www2.health.vic.gov.au/public-health/drugs-and-poisons/medicinal-cannabis/frequently-asked-questions, September 15, 2020.
78. *Treatment.* Multiple Sclerosis Australia. January 2018. Retrieved from https://www.ms.org.au/attachments/treatments-january-2018/treatment-sativex.aspx September 15, 2020.
79. Jennifer Nichols and Robert Blackmore, *Medicinal cannabis farm begins production vowing a duty of care to Australian patients.* ABC News, November 8, 2018. Retrieved on October 6, 2020 from https://www.abc.net.au/news/rural/2018-11-08/medifarm-medicinal-marijuana-first-plants-in-queensland/10476808
80. Dwight Blake, *Marijuana Tax Act of 1937: What you need to know.* American Marijuana, January 13, 2020. Retrieved September 17, 2020 from https://americanmarijuana.org/marijuana-tax-act-of-1937/
81. *The Australian Marijuana Grower's Guide.* Otter Publications, Redfern NSW (1996).
82. John Jiggens, *Marijuana Australiana: Cannabis use, Popular Culture and the Americanisation of Drugs Policy in Australia.* Self-published.
83. T. Makkai, I. McAllister, (1997). *Marijuana in Australia: Patterns and attitudes.* Looking Glass Press, Canberra.
84. D McDonald, R Moore, J. Norberry, G Wardlaw, & N. Ballenden, (1994). *Legislative options for cannabis in Australia.* Australian Government Publishing Service, Canberra.
85. J McLaren, R P Mattick, (2006). *Cannabis in Australia: Use, supply, harms, and* responses Monograph series No. 57. Report prepared for Drug Strategy Branch, Australian Government Department of Health and Ageing Drug and Alcohol Research Centre, University of New South Wales.
86. A Campbell, (2001). *The Australian Illicit Drug Guide: Every person's guide to illicit drugs – Their use, effects and history, treatment options and legal penalties.* Black Inc. National Library of Australian Cataloguing.
87. J Jiggens, (2007) In a Time of Murder – The Murder of Don Mackay, *StickyPoint Magazine,* Issue 02

88. Martin Booth (June 2005). *Cannabis: A History.* Picador.
89. Stephen Russell, *Hemp food legal from Sunday.* SBS, November 9, 2017. Retrieved September 18, 2020, from https://www.sbs.com.au/food/article/2017/11/09/hemp-food-legal-sunday
90. Tamika Seeto, *Medicinal Cannabis in Australia: Health Insurance.* Canstar, July 2, 2020. Retrieved September 15, 2020 from https://www.canstar.com.au/health-insurance/medicinal-marijuana-australia/
91. *Medicinal Cannabis Compassionate Use Scheme.* Centre for Medicinal Cannabis Research and Innovation. Retrieved September 18, 2020 from https://www.medicinalcannabis.nsw.gov.au/patients/medicinal-cannabis-compassionate-use-scheme
92. *Tests show potential for medicinal cannabis to kill cancer cells.* University News. University of Newcastle, July 20, 2020. Retrieved September 20, 2020 from https://www.newcastle.edu.au/newsroom/featured/tests-show-potential-for-medicinal-cannabis-to-kill-cancer-cells
93. *Guidance for the use of medicinal cannabis in Australia: Patient information.* Version 1, December 2017. Retrieved September 21, 2020 from https://www.tga.gov.au/publication/guidance-use-medicinal-cannabis-australia-patient-information
94. *Guidance for the use of medicinal cannabis in Australia: Patient information.* Version 1, December 2017. Retrieved September 21, 2020 from https://www.tga.gov.au/publication/guidance-use-medicinal-cannabis-australia-patient-information
95. *Biobran MGN-3 – An Overview.* BioBran.org. Retrieved September 20, 2020 from https://www.biobran.org/overview

www.ingramcontent.com/pod-product-compliance
Lightning Source LLC
Chambersburg PA
CBHW040241130526
44590CB00049B/4055